Don't Tell The Patient

Behind the Drug Safety Net

Don't Tell The Patient
Behind the Drug Safety Net

Bill Inman

HIGHLAND PARK PRODUCTIONS

For publishing information and US ordering:

Highland Park Productions

P.O.Box 41-1462

Los Angeles

California 90041-8462

HighlandPP@AOL.com

www.highlandpp.com

For UK ordering:

Highland Park Productions

P.O.Box 51

Bishops Waltham

Hampshire SO32-1YA

Copyright William Inman ©1999

The right of William Inman to be identified as the author of this book has been asserted in accordance with the United Kingdom Copyright, Designs and Patents Act 1988.

ISBN 0-9675812-0-6 (Hardbound)

Library of Congress Catalog Card Number 99-96417

Printed in the United States of America

Graphic Design by elle + elle, Los Angeles

Don't Tell The Patient, Behind the Drug Safety Net is a First Edition.

1 2 3 4 5 6 7 8 9 10

This book is dedicated to my wife June and my daughters, Stella, Rosemary and Charlotte and to many loyal colleagues who have supported me through the years.

Contents

Preface

This book is a semi-biographical "insider" account of my thirty years work in drug safety. Among other revelations it uncovers a serious and continuing scandal involving National Health Service (NHS) patients. Without their permission or any warning about possible risks, many of them have been treated with recently introduced drugs by GPs who receive substantial payments from drug companies under the pretext that they are taking part in research. The Department of Health has failed to stop this unethical practice.

Most clinical trials are controlled by company medical departments maintaining the highest ethical standards. Much of my work would have been impossible without the co-operation of their doctors and substantial "no-strings" support from medical department budgets. Once a new drug has been marketed, however, it is controlled by salesmen whose motivation is rather different. After marketing, the medical departments exert little or no control although they may have to "carry the can" to protect the company if something goes wrong.

The story of how I recovered from a near-fatal attack of polio contracted as a medical student at the age of twenty-one, half a century ago, and the fulfilling career that followed in spite of severe residual disability will be told in another book.[1] It is extremely unlikely that I would have found myself dedicated to work in drug safety if I had not to spend almost all of my adult life in a wheelchair.

From student in 1947 to retirement in 1994, my career spans some of the most exciting advances in the history of medicine and surgery, including the development of most of the drugs in use today. Aspirin, insulin and morphine are examples of the relatively few important exceptions and it is difficult to imagine practising medicine if these three drugs had not been discovered. There are more discoveries that I shall not be around to wonder at, such as the selective repair of chromosomes. Currently incurable conditions such as schizophrenia, Alzheimer's Disease, multiple sclerosis and many cancers may yield to new technology. Much of the conquest or amelioration of diseases that were either badly treated or untreatable when I became a medical student is to the credit of the pharmaceutical industry. However, success has not been achieved without accidents. I could not have guessed that the thalidomide disaster would focus my career on drug safety research or that I would spend most of my working life "Behind the Drug Safety Net". I became totally absorbed developing the only two drug-safety monitoring schemes currently operating on a national scale in the United Kingdom.

Each of the four phases of my working life has provided a different perspective on drug safety. I enjoyed a short spell in hospital medicine at a time when the side-effects of the rather small number of drugs we used were fairly well known. It was short because few career opportunities in clinical medicine were open to a young doctor who had gone through medical school in a wheelchair. Next I was employed as a medical adviser in the pharmaceutical industry, a second career that was interrupted after a few years by the thalidomide disaster and an invitation from Sir Derrick Dunlop, the first Chairman of the Committee on Safety of Drugs (CSD), to start the national early warning system for detecting adverse drug reactions, usually referred to as the "yellow card system." In spite of the constraints on scientific work within the civil service, I was able to conduct the first epidemiological study to produce evidence that the pill sometimes caused fatal thrombosis and an even more important study that led directly to the safer "Mini Pill."

The yellow card scheme uncovered many previously unrecognised problems. Its location within the Department of Health, however, was unfortunate because of the near impossibility of conducting research for an independent committee and serving the "establishment" at the same time. I shall give several examples of how the credibility of the Committee and the Department of Health was damaged because people tried, as indeed they continue to try, to mix science with politics and scientists with health-care managers.

In 1971, when the Medicines Act of 1968 became effective, a Licensing Authority was established and the secretariat of the Committee on Safety of Drugs was absorbed into it. The word "Drugs" was thought to be too emotive so we became the Committee on Safety of Medicines (CSM). From 1971 relations with the industry tended to become adversarial. Both sides were represented by doctor-advocates and I soon found myself unable to tolerate the compromise and expediency that this entailed. Internal confrontations between scientific and lay civil servants were also becoming more frequent. It was obvious that any fundamental progress in safety monitoring would only be achieved by moving to an environment in which one would be free to discuss and publish the results of one's research. It was quite improper for results to be massaged by officials into something they thought might be consistent with a departmental policy that would please the Minister of the day. A major disaster with a heart drug called Eraldin that had not been predicted by pre-marketing investigations and was not detected by the yellow cards, led me to my fourth career as founder and Director of the Drug Safety Research Unit (DSRU) at the University of Southampton. Here I developed the second national scheme for monitoring drug safety known as Prescription-Event Monitoring (PEM). The DSRU is managed by the Drug Safety Research

Trust as a non-profit charity independent of the government and the pharmaceutical industry. Its policies and rules described in this book are those that were in place up to the time of my retirement as Founder Director in 1994.

I am the only survivor of the original medical secretariat appointed to serve Sir Derrick Dunlop's Committee on Safety of Drugs (CSD) in 1964. I had many enjoyable discussions with him during those early months and we had both been concerned that it would be difficult, if not impossible, to be effective and loyal to a scientifically independent body and to political masters at the same time. We would almost certainly uncover some hazards that the Department would find hard to handle. We might have to change our minds as perceived risks melted away or the case against a drug strengthened as new data accumulated. Once a Minister has made a statement that has caught the attention of the public, officials would insist that significant changes in emphasis or "U-turns" had to be avoided at all costs even if the new evidence showed that the statement at the time was wrong. Experience with the Pill and the whooping-cough vaccine subsequently proved how accurate our predictions had been.

My story climaxed in a ten-year struggle against the exploitation of patients' trust in their doctors by pharmaceutical companies that used the need to monitor new drugs as a sales ploy. Under the guise of "Post-marketing Surveillance" (PMS) some doctors are fooled into believing that they are taking part in research and are paid to prescribe new drugs on ordinary NHS prescription forms. The patients are not volunteers and no explanation for change of treatment may be given. This is a prostitution of prescribing practice that has been largely unchallenged by successive governments because of the financial and employment consequences to the industry. My efforts fell a long way short of success and the main objective of this book is to draw public attention to this practice in the hope that others may take appropriate action.

During my thirty years in drug safety work I sometimes met with per-
versity and intellectual dishonesty that were far worse than any that I
could possibly have anticipated when I entered the drug-safety field. I
shall show how some people sought to undermine my efforts to expose
the group of doctors who are accepting substantial payments to prescribe new drugs of dubious efficacy and unknown safety. Skeletons will
be uncovered in several cupboards and some readers may be quite disturbed by them.

This is not a scientific book for a medical audience, nor is it a com-
prehensive historical account of all the hard work by the various independent committees and professional groups to improve drug safety after
the thalidomide disaster. A net may be described as many holes held
together by string. Sometimes it catches a fish. Sometimes the holes are
too big and a fish gets through. Big pharmaceutical fishes may become
very smelly very rapidly. With the help of dedicated staff and a forgiving
wife and family, I developed both national safety nets. This book explains
some of the activities which went on behind the scenes that the authorities would prefer you not to know about, and why some of the holes in
the net are still as large as they were thirty years ago.

I have tried to explain the nature of some of the problems such as
thrombosis in women using oral contraceptives without too much technical jargon. Occasionally I quote figures to show the scale of the problems that arose. Technical details and statistics may be unpalatable for
some readers but most will be interested in the possible effects of the
piece of paper they take away from the doctor's office. We have all been
patients at one time or another and will all be patients again. Brand or
trade names start with a capital letter to distinguish them from the longer
scientific names. I have tended to refer to patients as "her" simply because
twice as many prescriptions are written for women as for men and
because women live longer. Similarly, when referring to doctors, I have

tended to use "him" because they outnumber women in most branches of medicine.

Finally, although I hope those I have left behind will maintain the principles I tried to establish and will continue to fight the abuses I have described, the views I have expressed in this book are entirely my own.

Southampton, England   July 1999

Acknowledgements

My wife June corrected numerous drafts and reminded me how to spell and punctuate, something that I had left to secretaries for more than forty years. But this task was trivial when compared with the support she gave me in my work in drug safety monitoring for more than thirty years. For half this time she had to play second fiddle to the Committee on Safety of Medicines and the Department of Health and for the other half to the Drug Safety Research Unit, both of which demanded my total attention and cost many of life's normal 'perks' such as family holidays. June received no public recognition, but without her support the first system might have disappeared and the second would not have got off the ground.

My original plan was to combine the story of a career in drug safety studies with an autobiographical account of my life as a student and doctor in a wheelchair and its many unusual and often amusing predicaments. Sincere thanks go to Betty Beaty whose experience as a writer and advice about the risk of losing one's readers if they are asked to flit from topic to topic, steered me to write two books. *Feeling Better Doctor?* will be ready soon. Several family members and friends have read the manuscript and offered helpful suggestions. I am particularly grateful to my daughter Charlotte of Highland Park Productions.

1 Before Thalidomide

I believe I revealed my ambition to become a doctor when I was only nine years old and, despite distractions such as wanting to be a Spitfire pilot, my resolve persisted throughout my school life and the war and I "went up" to Gonville and Caius College, Cambridge, to start my medical career in 1947. After three years' study of anatomy, physiology, pathology and allied subjects, and an enjoyable social life, I applied for a place at St. Thomas's Hospital for my clinical training. This plan was frustrated, however, when I developed a severe case of infantile paralysis, inconveniently coinciding with the middle of the examinations in 1950. After a short spell in an "iron lung," I spent a few months in orthopaedic hospitals and struggled with full-length leg-irons (callipers) attached to a leather and metal contraption called a "pelvic band." It had sliding catches that enabled me to sit down but had to be locked rigidly when I stood up so that I had to swing my body and legs in one piece, hanging from my crutches. Walking was clearly going to be impracticable, so I left hospital much earlier than predicted and rapidly adapted to life in a wheelchair. I acquired a car with hand-controls, an Austin *A 90 Atlantic* convertible capable of a "Ton" (100 miles per hour). It was hardly the most appropriate choice for a disabled driver, but it had huge doors that made it easy for me to get my folding wheelchair into it unaided. Having booked a driving test before the car was delivered, I learned how to use hand controls by driving my parents to Scarborough for the weekend.

They were more confident in my ability than I was, but the journey was without incident and the following Monday morning I passed the test. I started working for Imperial Chemical Pharmaceuticals Ltd. (ICP) a week later. I have described my experience of living with and overcoming severe disability in *Feeling Better Doctor?* that I hope to publish shortly.[1] What follows in this first chapter is merely a brief summary of the next fourteen years leading to the start of my career "behind the safety net."

Imperial Chemical Industries' (ICI) interest in drugs started in its Dyestuffs Division which had its headquarters at Blackley in the northern outskirts of Manchester. The new subsidiary, Imperial Chemical Pharmaceuticals Ltd. (ICP) had offices in Wilmslow, Cheshire, and was rapidly establishing its products in several areas of medicine. At the time I joined it was about to introduce a new anaesthetic agent, halothane, that would replace chloroform or the highly inflammable ether that had put me and my two brothers to sleep during a tonsillectomy session at a cottage hospital during the war. It had developed one of the earliest sulphonamide anti-bacterials and its range of products included peni-cillin, a drug for epilepsy called primidone and antiseptics such as cetrim-ide. The company was also a leader in the development of drugs for trop-ical diseases. Paludrine had played a vital role in the control of malaria among troops fighting in the Far East. Several other anti-malarial and anti-leprosy drugs were currently under trial. Two large adjacent houses in Wilmslow in Cheshire, Fulshaw Hall and Harefield Hall, accommodated the medical and administrative departments. New research facilities were planned at Alderley Park near Macclesfield which would later become one of the largest pharmaceutical research complexes in Europe.

I was employed as a technical abstractor in the Medical Department and as the main building had no lift, my office was in a prefabricated building in the kitchen garden at Harefield. As a recruit to "Reviews and Abstracts," my job was to prepare a one or two-page précis of any article about the company's products that had appeared in the world medical and veterinary journals, as well as for drugs produced by rival companies that might be of interest to ICP's research or commercial departments. I also prepared summaries of internal research papers to be used in briefing the company's commercial staff. The work was interesting and taught me the importance of clear presentation and brevity. It was often necessary to summarise a document running to fifty pages into no more than two. The ability to extract "key" information and to discard unnecessary details was to prove invaluable throughout my subsequent career. "Reviews and Abstracts" ran parallel with a complementary but smaller Intelligence Section run by a former King's Messenger, Sir John Chichester. His responsibility was to scan the newspapers and trade journals for information that was useful to the commercial side of the management. The two sections provided a service for the company similar to that nowadays fulfilled by abstracting journals and computer databases. The Medical Department comprised three doctors and was headed by an anaesthetist, Dr. Ben Wevill, assisted by Alex Stewart and Kenneth Green. One day, after I had been working for the company for about nine months, Dr. Wevill called me to his office and made what at first seemed an extraordinary proposal. Wheelchair or not, he insisted, I should return to medicine! He had been impressed by my work, but it was a dead-end job. He believed it was possible to qualify in medicine entirely in a wheelchair and suggested that I should think it over and see him again in a week or so. I was also encouraged to consider this change of plan by the Chairman, Sam Howard, and the Managing Director, Dermot Carey.

It was now two years from my attack of polio. Except for my inability to walk I was enjoying a surprisingly normal life. With my A 90 I could travel anywhere in the country. My arms and hands were quite strong, although I had lost some of the fine movements of my fingers and hand-writing was difficult; I had learned to type. I could use tools almost normally and could jack up the car and change a wheel without help while sitting in my wheelchair. Although access to many public buildings and most private houses was difficult, I realised that all hospitals would have lifts. I also enjoyed many recreational activities. Having been a keen field-sportsman I could again take my place in a line of guns at a game shoot and manipulate my chair over rough ground. I had already completed my preliminary studies of anatomy and physiology before being stricken by polio, though I would have to retake some of the exams. As a pre-clinical student I could see no reason why I should not learn to examine and treat patients and practise in any medical speciality where mobility was not a prime consideration. Obviously general practice or surgery would be impossible but there were numerous other possibilities such as laboratory medicine, dermatology, psychiatry, or public health.

I drove to London to meet the Dean of Medicine at St. Thomas's Hospital, Dr. MacSweeney, who had originally offered me a place in 1950. MacSweeney took one look at me and explained there was not the slightest chance that I could cope with the architecture of St. Thomas's or its medical school. He believed, however, that the Secretary of the Medical School, Dr. A. L. Crockford, had some helpful ideas. "Crock", as he was known to the students, was a delightful man, unusually distinguished by having won a Military Cross in the first world war and a Distinguished Service Order in the second. He had been Secretary of the Medical School and a tutor for four years and I was sorry he would not be supervising me if I resumed my career. Crockford picked up the phone and had a long conversation with John Woodcock, Secretary of the postgraduate medical school at Cambridge, while I listened, impressed by his total grasp of my situation. Although Cambridge did not have a teaching hospital the Regius Professor of Physic, Sir Lionel Whitby, had always cherished an ambition to start one at Addenbrooke's Hospital to compete with the school in Oxford. In those days, after completing their pre-clinical studies of anatomy and physiology and armed with a B.A.Cantab., graduates moved to a teaching hospital in London or the provinces to learn their art with the help of real patients. Those who wished to take the University Degree returned to Cambridge three years later for their final qualifying examinations. I presented a challenge and an opportunity to fulfil Lionel Whitby's dream. I would receive no formal training, but could depend on the consultants and their registrars for informal guidance and would enjoy the great advantage of a large and busy city hospital to myself! Sadly, Whitby died of cancer soon after I started and further development of the school was delayed for many years. I was to have the distinction of being the first student to complete my clinical studies entirely at Addenbrooke's and to qualify as a doctor at the new "medical school" several years before it became one! Two years later an able-bodied student, Douglas Perkins, succeeded in qualifying by the same route. But I am jumping ahead of my story.

I reported back to Dr. Wevill that my initial qualms had largely evaporated. He promised that if the project should turn out to be too difficult, the Company would keep a job open for me. He then went even further and suggested that after I had got my medical degree and some clinical experience there would be a job for me in the Medical Department should I decide that other avenues were impracticable or unattractive. I owe an immense debt of gratitude to Ben Wevill, Alex Stewart and Ken Green for their long-sightedness and readiness to cover my line of retreat.

In 1952 I left ICP and returned to Cambridge. It was to become the focal point of my life for nearly seven years. I found a flat at Madingley Hall, a large mansion about three miles from Cambridge, used by the University as a hall of residence for extra-mural students. Many of the residents were attending "Devonshire Courses" for overseas students or working for their PhD. The Hall was always filled with interesting people, several of whom became life-long friends. I spent a fairly relaxed six months revising for the exams that I had failed to complete when I went down with polio and I passed them quite easily. As handwriting was impossible I was allowed to type my papers in a side room.

As the only student at Addenbrooke's Hospital and without any formal lectures, I learned my medicine by practical experience during consultants' ward-rounds and informal sessions with the registrars and junior housemen, and by studying textbooks in the evenings. I had a 280-bed hospital entirely to myself, a big advantage over a teaching hospital where there are several students per bed. Ward-rounds were often attended by local general practitioners and overseas doctors and after "shadowing" the registrars and housemen for a few weeks, learning by example how to examine patients and record their "histories," I was invited to introduce the cases that I had "clerked." I soon found that the wheelchair put me at little disadvantage in the wards, indeed it often helped me to establish a rapport with patients who would frequently enquire—"feeling better Doctor?" I was attached to one of the three medical firms headed by Dr. Leslie Cole, a general physician with a special interest in the heart. It was he who had made the decision to release me from the iron lung three years earlier. I also attended ward rounds by Dr. Laurence Martin, a general physician who was also a distinguished endocrinologist. Each of the three medical firms admitted patients for one week in turn. Being involved with almost all admissions by Dr. Cole's firm, I was able to follow the whole process of diagnosis and treatment of about one third of all the "general" medical admissions. "General" excluded patients admitted to special departments such as paediatrics or psychiatry; that would come later. I still had time to study in the pathology laboratories or other special departments and to sit in with consultants during their out-patient sessions. I was encouraged to play all the roles of the junior doctors and, with so much practice, soon became skilful in setting up transfusions and performing lumbar-punctures and other procedures. I worked late into the night during the weeks "on take" for medical emergencies. This was the sharp end of medicine and the most exciting.

Leslie Cole was a small, scholarly and immensely polite man who would never humiliate a student or "score points" off a houseman in front of an audience. "What you need, Inman, is a high index of suspicion." I never forgot his advice to look for the unusual and to question my own and even the experts' diagnoses, while remembering at the same time his other slogan that "common things occur commonly"; in other words never to allow oneself to be carried away by the "small print." Leslie Cole's Senior Registrar was John Wedgwood, a descendent of the founder of the famous Staffordshire pottery. John generously gave up his time to teach me in the ward office or at the bedside, as did a part-time consultant in haematology, John Marks, who was also the first Medical Director of the United Kingdom subsidiary of Roche, the large Swiss pharmaceutical company. Long before my final examinations, John suggested that I might like to join him as his assistant in the company's new medical department after I had qualified. I have often wondered if my life would have taken an entirely different course had I taken up his kind offer.

After completing my "clinical clerking" I became a "surgical dresser" to one of the three general surgical firms headed by John Withycombe, who specialised in urology. I took histories and examined most of the general surgical cases admitted to the hospital every third week when Withycombe's firm was "on take" for emergencies, as well as waiting-list cases admitted when beds became available. This still left me with ample time to attend surgical outpatients or to work in the casualty department. John Withycombe's Australian registrar, Des Cooper, taught me most of my surgery. The hospital carpenter constructed a seat-raiser comprising a wooden box with a raised backrest that enabled me to sit at "standing" height and assist at operations. It was fitted with a safety belt to prevent me falling onto (or into) the patient during the operation! I assisted Des at procedures such as the removal of a stomach or gallbladder, and became adept at "swabbing, sucking and suturing" and holding heavy retractors for long periods. The casualty department was also a rich source of practical experience in both medicine and surgery. Many hours were spent cleaning and stitching wounds and applying plaster bandages to fractures. Concurrent with my work on the wards I was instructed in pathology by Basil Herbertson, Granville Naylor and Michael Stoker, with demonstrations in the post-mortem room by Austin Gresham. The wheel-chair, however, precluded doing post-mortems myself, for which I was somewhat relieved.

I received informal teaching in the eye department from Mr. Recordon and in ear nose and throat surgery from the Senior Registrar, Claude Eastes. Arthur Rook taught me dermatology, and I did a few sessions at Fulbourn Mental Hospital with Dr. Russell Davies, in the paediatric department with Douglas Gairdner and in other specialised departments such as orthopaedics and ophthalmology. Bill Grundy gave me special tuition in pharmacology, the study of drugs, that turned out to be partic-ularly appropriate in view of the career I was eventually to follow. Most of those who made it possible for me to qualify as a doctor have died, but it is a privilege to acknowledge their generous help.

The greatest physical challenge was obstetrics and although some people doubted my ability to deliver the twenty babies required to obtain a signature in the "grey book" in which progress through medical school was recorded, this turned out to be much too pessimistic. (Later, some pessimists thought I was unlikely to learn to fly gliders and were to be proved equally wrong when I went solo and won a cup as the best pupil pilot). Students were expected to deliver five babies under close supervi-sion in a teaching hospital, and then to accompany a midwife to attend fifteen more in the district hospitals or the patients' own homes. I was given a room at the Mill Road Maternity Hospital and spent an enjoyable two months delivering a total of fifty-six infants from fifty-five deliveries (one set of twins). Although nowadays most women are delivered in the more natural semi-reclining or squatting position, in the early '50s it was still usual to deliver them lying on their left side with a nurse holding up the right leg. This suited me well.

By the summer of 1956 I was on the last lap before the finals. My main problem was that I was only able to write legibly for a few minutes at a time and would have to type all my papers. Few examination questions are entirely novel and the important ones recur frequently. I had therefore typed carefully prepared answers to all the questions that had been set during the past ten years, practising my typing at the same time. My answers were brief and "examiner-friendly" and exactly the length that I knew I could type comfortably in the time available. The lessons I had learned in "Reviews and Abstracts" were invaluable. I had worked hard and played hard and I approached the final test with a fair measure of confidence. I was in good physical and mental shape. Rather than spend the last few days in feverish revision, I took the week off to stay with my parents on the south coast.

The papers and vivas presented no serious problems and on December 18th 1956, I was proud to learn on the telephone that I had qualified as a Bachelor of Medicine and Surgery of Cambridge University. The polio had cost three years and my legs. My former Tutor, Hubert Tunnicliffe, called to congratulate me and passed on the comments of the examiners. Several had expressed the wish that all students typed their papers. He also told me that, although marks are not published, I had been one of the first small handful of candidates in every subject. Laurence Martin immediately invited me to be his houseman and the General Medical Council agreed that, instead of doing one medical and one surgical job during my first year, I would be allowed to do two consecutive medical jobs to satisfy their requirements for full registration. Clearly they appreciated that I was unlikely to pose a threat to public safety as a surgeon.

The transition from student to junior doctor proved to be far less difficult than I had anticipated. I started in my first medical post as house physician to Laurence Martin at the end of January 1957. I was working with familiar people doing all the things I had done before, but with greater responsibility. Unlike most newly qualified doctors, I had already performed all the routine procedures such as setting up transfusions, lumbar punctures and minor surgery on dozens of occasions, but now I was also responsible for ordering all the appropriate investigations and justifying their cost, planning the ward rounds, finding beds for emergency cases and prescribing drugs. Throughout this period I do not recall any occasion in which my wheelchair was more than a minor inconvenience in the ward, although one demented patient did succeed in kicking me out of it with a well-aimed blow to my head.

With the first appointment successfully completed, and because I was exempted from the surgical appointment, it was decided that I should take over a newly created post that was originally intended for a more senior doctor. I was to look after the beds belonging to a number of specialist departments that were scattered round the hospital. They included all the chest cases admitted by Dr. Martin Greenberg, a few beds belonging to Professor McCance, Head of the Department of Experimental Medicine, and patients with blood disorders and cancer receiving chemotherapy in the University Department of Haematology headed by Dr. Frank Hayhoe. I looked after thirty beds and the pace of the work was rather more leisurely than in my first job because most patients were admitted from the waiting list and few as emergencies. I worked with these groups for two and a half years but realised that I would soon have to make a fundamental decision. I had succeeded in qualifying in medicine and had completed my pre-registration jobs and the more senior resident post, but the range of career opportunities was limited. Difficult access to buildings would also preclude consultancies in general medicine where, in those days, it was usual to make home visits to patients. General practice was even more impossible. I was not keen on psychiatry or dermatology. A whole range of laboratory specialities such as biochemistry or bacteriology was available but not very appealing either. The more I thought about the future and discussed it with colleagues, the more sensible seemed the original proposal by Ben Wevill that a worthwhile career could be based on pharmaceutical medicine. New and exciting discoveries were being made. The industry was expanding as the National Health Service created a vast and assured market for drugs. From my brief encounter in 1951, I realised I would have to be careful to avoid becoming a medically qualified "super-rep" and I had qualms about some of the sales practises that I had encountered. I had been unhappy about the amount of entertaining involved in persuading doctors to prescribe the company's drugs and I was particularly aware that immigrant doctors working in unattractive city practices were considered by the company "reps" to be "soft targets" for somewhat questionable promotional techniques. I shall have more to say about this towards the end of this book. On the positive side, ICI Pharmaceuticals was a research-based company and had a strong medical department: I decided to return.

As the pharmaceutical industry was to become such an important part of my life I shall briefly describe its origins in the dyestuffs industry. Traditionally, dyestuffs had been extracted from plants such as indigo or madder but the colours tended to be inconsistent and often faded after washing or exposure to sunlight. In 1856, W.H. Perkin, who was looking for a method to synthesise quinine, was the first to produce and market a reliable synthetic dye produced from a coal-tar derivative called aniline. At that time Britain had the world's largest textile industry and it also had an almost inexhaustible supply of coal-tar as a waste product of gas production. It might have been expected that Britain would also rapidly establish world leadership in dyestuffs production and the development of other organic chemicals including drugs. In the second half of the nineteenth century, however, Germany rapidly became the dominant power in the chemical, explosives and dyestuffs industries. By the outbreak of the First World War it had achieved a virtual monopoly in dyestuffs, accounting for more than eighty percent of world production, compared with a derisory three percent achieved by Great Britain. With the lead captured by Germany, the textile industry had to turn to it to supply dyestuffs more cheaply and efficiently than the eleven small British coal-tar dye factories were able to do. Inevitably, Germany also took the lead in the diversification of dyestuffs into synthetic rubber, photographic chemicals and drugs. These were lost opportunities that can be attributed to defects in the British education system.[2]

For three centuries Britain suffered economically and socially because the products of its inventiveness had been crushed by its educational system, dominated by clergymen and classicists with their contempt for "trade." In their defence it should be said that at least their pupils left school numerate, able to spell and with hand-writing that was worth reading, but there was a profound shortage of scientists and engineers. A predominantly non-agricultural nation cannot earn enough to enjoy the richness of its culture if its leaders, and particularly its public servants who manipulate resources, are brought up on a diet of Shakespeare and Shelley rather than physics and chemistry. The best technical people do not make a career in the civil service unless co-opted from outside as "advisers" to cope with some emergency, in which event, as we shall see repeatedly in later chapters, they are kept "on tap," but not "on top." Technical experts are better paid elsewhere. Perhaps the most tragic example (and the history of the British dyestuffs industry is another one) of the lack of foresight by government was the development of the jet engine that Frank Whittle patented in 1932 but was not built until 1937 and first flown, after nearly two years of war, in May 1941. With adequate support from a civil service that listened to its scientists and engineers, the first British jet fighters would have flown at least four years earlier, well before the outbreak of war; had they done so, it is possible that Hitler might not have risked starting it. Germany had jet aircraft in the air two years before the British, and after the war, when the Ministry cancelled the programme that would almost certainly have enabled Britain to be the first to break the sound barrier, the honour went to the Bell company in the United States. The design of the Bell 100 had been copied from plans that had been shared with the Americans by the Miles company of Britain. It was immediately declared by the Pentagon to be state secret and treated them as the United States' exclusive property.

That Britain's dyestuffs industry survived into the twentieth century may be attributed to one man – and he was not British. Ivan Levinstein (1845-1916) was a German Jew who came to Lancashire in 1864 to seek his fortune. He founded Levinstein Ltd. of Blackley near Manchester at the age of only nineteen! Recognising the reasons behind the inferiority of the UK industry in comparison with Germany he did his best to foster technical education in the region. He became a governor of Owens College in Manchester in the hope of encouraging the training of young scientists, but in spite of this initiative he had to turn to German banks for what he called "educated money." From the turn of the century his firm began to prosper and absorb other companies and his son Herbert began to recruit and train good quality scientific staff. Ivan's son was able to claim with some justification that his father had "saved the British dyestuffs industry."

In 1911, Gesellschaft für chemische Industrie in Basel, better known as CIBA, bought the small rival Clayton Aniline Company in Manchester. About the same time the German Hoechst company set up a subsidiary company in Ellesmere Port in Cheshire. These and other continental countries were poised to become the world's leading drug manufacturers. When the war broke out, the Levinsteins instantly gained an advantage, producing enough khaki to dye the uniforms for nine million men! They partnered with CIBA who provided vital intermediates without letting any similar materials cross the Swiss border into Germany. The war provided the opportunity needed by the British dyestuffs industry to redress the earlier imbalance. Levinstein was allowed by the government to buy the German Hoechst plant at Ellesmere Port. In November 1917 Harry McGowan, the future chairman of ICI, joined the Board of Levinstein. After demobilisation in 1919 my father, who was to become the Chairman of ICI's largest division, formerly Brunner Mond Ltd and later the Alkali Division, began work as a research chemist in the United Alkali Company (UAC) laboratories at Widnes, one of several companies amalgamating to form ICI in 1926.

In 1919 the British Dyestuffs Corporation Ltd (BDC) was formed as a holding company, with Levinsteins and British Dyes as its main sub-sidiaries. Also about this time, however, the development of the dyestuffs element of the chemical industry started to slow down. British production of dyes exceeded demand because of the post-war recovery of German industry. The British government then stepped into the arena and from 1919 to 1926 became a majority shareholder in BDC. This was govern-ment's first attempt to control a major industrial enterprise and, like most subsequent attempts at nationalisation, it failed miserably with massive loss of public funds. In 1926 the government sold its BDC shares to Nobel Industries which was incorporated into ICI the same year, perhaps one of the earliest examples of "privatisation."

ICI's interest in drug manufacture was concentrated in its dyestuffs division at Blackely in Manchester until it spawned I.C.Pharmaceuticals shortly before I first joined it in 1951. When I returned to Cheshire eight years later, the research laboratories employed a number of former dyestuffs chemists and toxicologists from Blackley and a large complex of research laboratories had been built at Mereside, South of Alderley Edge. The Company was now known as the Pharmaceuticals Division of ICI. Thirty years later it would become a major part of the new company, Zeneca, following the demerger of ICI.

Ben Wevill, whose wise advice had lead me to resume my career in medicine had moved up to the Board of the Company, and the head of the Medical Department was now Alex Stewart with Kenneth Green as his deputy. The third member of the department was a huge amiable man weighing more than twenty stone, Michael Mungavin, with whom I shared a room at Harefield Hall for a few months before the department was moved to Alderley Park. Michael had worked for some time in the Far East as a specialist in tropical medicine. Alex was a "canny Scott" and Ken (the brother of Nigel Green the actor) was a "laid back" character, both, in their quite different ways, ideal people to generate charisma among professional customers and their own staff. I am the only survivor of the four doctors who ran the medical department at the time I joined it in 1959. Shortly after there were three more recruits, Cecil Marsden, a dermatologist, Colin Downie, formerly the medical officer to Bristol University, and Jimmy Langtry who handled the company's trials in Latin-America. Each of us was responsible for several new products under development. Mine included drugs for epilepsy, reduction of cholesterol and anaemia, a range of dyes injected into blood vessels for diagnostic purposes, and drugs used in cancer chemotherapy.

One of the methods for studying the circulation of the blood, nowadays completely outdated, involved injecting dyes into the blood-stream and measuring the rate of their appearance in different parts of the body. The "circulation-time," for example, could be estimated by injecting dye into a vein in the arm and measuring how long it took to be detected by a photo-electric device clipped to the ear-lobe. It measured the output of the heart and the effects of abnormalities such as "holes in the heart." The dye, called Coomassie Blue after an obscure tribe from Kumasi in the Gold Coast (later Ghana), had been produced by ICI Dyestuffs Division because it was thought to be less toxic than other dyes such as Evans Blue. It was provided as a service to specialists and had no commercial future. Such products, however, created goodwill among senior professionals working in a wide variety of fields. Coomassie Blue was also my first introduction to my friend for thirty years, South African Jeff Thorpe, a larger-than-life character who became widely known and respected throughout the world of cardiology for his work on drugs that lowered the cholesterol, notably clofibrate, better known as Atromid. Jeff, who had started life as an engineer, seemed to have succeeded in squeezing several scientific and social lifetimes into one, including two wives and families. He was a bon viveur, a passable golfer and an undisputed world expert in fat-metabolism. Because of the huge potential market for a drug that would, hopefully, reduce mortality from coronary disease, Atromid became one of our major products. Jeff in his cups at the Blacksmith's Arms one day, told me - "For God's sake don't tell anybody, Bill, but there is a lot of bullshit being talked about Atromid's unique effect on the platelets. Aspirin will do exactly the same thing." Platelets are small fragments of cells that tend to stick on roughened surfaces such as wounds or the walls of damaged blood vessels, starting the process of blood-clotting. Like the proverbial elephant, I remembered everything in those days and it was no surprise, a quarter of a century later, when small doses of aspirin taken every day became a cheap and effective way of reducing mortality from disease of the coronary arteries. I shall refer later to some work I did that supported Jeff's hypothesis that many acidic organic compounds could have this effect.

The use of dyes to decide if tissues damaged by injury had retained sufficient blood-supply to survive led me to some very exciting and dramatic experiments. When a patient has been badly burnt it is not always easy to decide whether particular areas of skin are viable. If all the three layers of skin have been burnt (a "third degree" burn) the dead skin has to be removed and the burnt area covered with a graft. Round the margins of the burn, however, it is sometimes difficult to decide how much full-thickness destruction has occurred and this could have lead to more extensive removal than was necessary. Two plastic surgeons, Emlyn Lewis and Michael Tempest, working in Chepstow, used another ICI dye called disulphine blue, injected into a vein to determine the extent of tissue that would have to be removed. The dye would not pass into the dead skin. The method worked well but there was a problem. For several days the patient remained a rich shade of bluish-green! The "Green Men of Chepstow" as I called them could be disconcerting for relatives on visiting day if they had not been warned in advance. Besides determining the extent of a burn, the dye injections could also be used to assess the success of grafts.

The Green Men of Chepstow inspired me to look for other possible applications of dye-injection techniques in neurosurgery and orthopaedics. Henry Maslowski, a Manchester neurosurgeon, used the green dye to outline brain tumours. Normal brain tissue did not take up the dye while the tumour turned green. Disulphine blue was sometimes useful when treating cancer patients with another ICI product that I had been responsible for during its clinical trials. It was known as Epodyl and was injected directly into the artery that fed the tumour. After passing through the cancerous tissue, and hopefully killing the cells selectively, it was rapidly destroyed in the general circulation and produced less damage to the bone-marrow than other anti-cancer drugs used in those days.

The war in Korea was producing survivors who, thanks to great improvements in surgery and the treatment of shock, were being resuscitated and returned home, sometimes with horrific injuries. One problem was the disparity between the seemingly small amount of superficial damage done by penetrating bullet wounds and the enormous amount of internal damage. A high-velocity bullet could pass through the fleshy part of a man's thigh leaving clean entry and exit wounds and missing the thigh-bone by several centimetres and yet shatter it completely and tear major blood vessels and nerves that were well away from the bullet track. It was known that some nearly spent bullets may start to tumble as they pass through the tissue causing more damage than one would expect. This was not, however, the explanation for the massive damage often produced by bullets that passed through flesh without tumbling. The development of ultra-high speed X-ray cinematography had made it possible to "freeze" a bullet travelling through a gelatine block that simulated flesh. Penetrating at more than the speed of sound, the shock wave caused a large temporary cavity many times the diameter of the bullet.

I was invited one day to the secret experimental establishment at Porton Down to shoot some sheep! Of course I did not shoot any sheep myself and I had rather mixed feelings about the experiments, but having lost a good friend in Korea I strongly approved of the work they were doing. In any case, the sheep were anaesthetised before they were shot and were then killed by lethal injection. A rifle barrel was clamped to a trolley on rails at one end of the range and tested on a target. The anaesthetised animal was then set up lying on its back on a table with the legs extended and the thigh very precisely fixed in line with the target. Although the diameter of the bullet was less than six millimetres, it momentarily produced a cavity ninety millimetres in diameter. The dye displayed the extent of the residual damage very well.[3] The Porton workers concluded, however, that disulphine blue was not giving as good results as some other techniques they had tried. In more horrific experiments conducted by the US. Army at their equivalent establishment in Maryland, sheep were literally blasted by small charges of explosives and disulphine blue was used to assess the extent of the damage. They claimed that the dye technique seemed to be a more reliable method and would be particularly useful in people who had been blown up by land-mines.[4]

And so here I was, comfortably established in a secure and interesting job and married with two children: and then came thalidomide. Our tranquillity was about to be violently disturbed and the whole course of my career was to change for ever.

2 "Father of the Mini Pill"

In 1956, Dr. Mückter and his colleagues working for the German company, Chemie Grünenthal, synthesised a drug called thalidomide. It showed considerable promise as a sleeping tablet with few side-effects and had the great advantage of not having the lethal effects of barbiturates when taken in overdoses. Insomnia is a common symptom of depression and the risk of suicide with any sleeping tablet is a most important consideration in the management of depressive illness. The other major problem is the risk of "hangover" effects that might affect driving, the operation of machinery or other tasks requiring concentration. Barbiturate overdoses outnumbered all hospital admissions of attempted suicides that I had to deal with as a junior doctor in the mid-fifties. Dogs had survived quantities of thalidomide that were one thousand times the dose required to make them sleep and subsequently patients who had attempted suicide with thalidomide had survived doses of at least one hundred times the normal dose. There was no doubt that claims for safety, in this sense, were amply justified. The invention of thalidomide was a new venture for a company used to making cosmetics and household products that had little or no experience in the manufacture of pharmaceuticals. Chemie Grünenthal started to sell thalidomide in Germany in October 1957 under the name of Contergan, and in England the Distillers Company started to sell it under licence as Distaval. Among the claims for thalidomide were safety for both mother and child if it was used during pregnancy. There is now some suspicion that evidence sug-gesting that thalidomide might damage the nerves in the limbs of adults was available to Grünenthal in 1959. They may not have been sufficiently experienced to understand the significance of the early reports but they have been accused of deliberately ignoring them because of the threat to the commercial success of the drug. At that time there was no reliable way to protect the public from ignorance, incompetence or fraud.

In December 1961, the *Lancet* published a letter by Dr. William McBride of Sydney, Australia, pointing out that, while about one and a half percent of all babies are born with congenital abnormalities, almost twenty percent of those born to mothers who had taken thalidomide had abnormalities, including striking limb deformities.[5] Unfortunately, the letter appeared some considerable time after he wrote it, having first been rejected by another journal. Dr. Widukind Lenz, a Hamburg children's specialist, first voiced his suspicions about thalidomide at a meeting in November 1961 and later reported, as a comment on McBride's letter, that he had seen fifty-two babies with abnormalities whose mothers had taken thalidomide in early pregnancy.[6] Later estimates from Germany were between two and three thousand. In the United Kingdom, it was officially reported retrospectively that there had been three hundred and forty-nine malformed children (eighty-two were born dead) whose mothers had def-initely or probably taken thalidomide.[7]

This could easily have been a disaster for Imperial Chemical Pharmaceuticals (ICP) because we sold several products under licence from Dista, the distributors of thalidomide in the UK, but had very fortunately not added thalidomide to the ICP list. As an observer rather than a partic-ipant in this tragedy, I discussed various ways of monitoring new drugs with a number of colleagues, and in 1963 I wrote to the Department of Health to enquire about their plans to set up a scheme for scrutinising new drugs both before and after they had been marketed. I was quite surprised to receive a personal letter from Sir Derrick Dunlop, the Chairman of a newly created Committee on Safety of Drugs (CSD), inviting me to consider joining the Secretariat of his committee and to develop a national scheme for gathering and analysing reports of suspected adverse reactions to drugs.

Early in 1964 I was interviewed at Alexander Flemming House, the Headquarters of the Department of Health and Social Security, by Sir Derrick Dunlop and some senior officials including Dr. Dennis Cahal, the Head of the medical secretariat and Wilfred Turner, the Secretary to the CSD. They had already made elaborate plans for testing drugs in animals and man before releasing them on the market and they were concerned about the lack of any reliable means for preventing further accidents when they were sold for general use. They asked for my ideas for monitoring new drugs. I recognised that it would always be impossible to avoid unforeseen accidents, but their scale when they did occur might be reduced if some form of early warning scheme could be devised. Obviously, the first line of defence was to collect all the information obtained by the manufacturers during their experiments in laboratory animals and in the early clinical trials. However, the small number of patients that can be assembled for most pre-marketing clinical trials will only reveal events that are so common that the hazard they present makes it unlikely that the drug company will proceed with a marketing licence application. Less common but nevertheless very important effects will often not be detected. For example, except by chance, a trial on one hundred patients could not be expected to detect a harmful reaction that only affected one patient in a thousand. I believed that it was vitally important to invite all doctors to report any events that they suspected might have been caused by new drugs and, indeed, this conclusion had already been reached by the committee. I was not happy, however, that such a system would be reliable unless there was also some means of following up individual cases to obtain details that might confirm that a drug was the cause. I proposed that a team of medically qualified field officers should be appointed to follow up the reports by visiting the doctors and discussing their reports at first hand.

The interviewing panel seemed to like what they heard and offered me a post as Medical Officer on the spot. Keen though I was, I felt that the post was too junior. I was asked to leave the room and was called back about three minutes later to be offered the job as Senior Medical Officer (SMO). There was little financial advantage and no company car, but I saw an interesting challenge and I indicated that I would almost certainly accept. I asked for a week to make up my mind and discuss it with my family. I returned to Cheshire to break the news to Ken Green and I asked ICI to release me as soon as possible. Again the company showed exemplary generosity and offered to re-employ me if the proposed scheme should fail or the Dunlop Committee was wound up. ICI agreed to release me as soon as I could find a house and move the family.

The move to London involved far more than a change of job. For the last fourteen years I had spent my time adapting to my disability, qualifying in medicine, achieving as near-normal a life-style as possible, holding down a job and raising a family. The new venture was decidedly risky. The government might fail to secure co-operation from the medical profession. Doctors might see reporting of adverse reactions as an admission of guilt for having harmed a patient. The post that I had been offered was a temporary one, although I was assured that it would automatically be made permanent or, in civil service parlance, "established," in about a year. On the positive side I now had an opportunity to do something that had never been done before in the United Kingdom and with only partial success in other countries. My new work was directly relevant to the safety of millions of people.

I started on September 1, 1964, living in an hotel in London during the week and the family moved to Hever in Kent in October. I could drive to work in London in just over one hour each way (a journey that was often to take over two hours each way when I left in 1980, an intrusion on life that had become unacceptable). The CSD's office was in Queen Anne's Mansions, since demolished, on the corner of Petty France and Queen Street, not far from Westminster Abbey. I had a large airy room on the tenth floor overlooking Petty France where I could watch the first Boeing 747s hanging, seemingly almost motionless, in the air beyond the Army and Navy Stores, as they flew along the Thames on their final approach to Heathrow sixteen miles to the West. My room was No.1007, but some wag had removed the first figure, so as "007," the "James Bond of drug safety," I spent the most enjoyable first five of the sixteen years that I was to work in London.

The CSD met every month and was served by three sub-committees that also met every month. Head of the permanent secretariat was Dr. Dennis Cahal. The Toxicity Sub-committee chaired by Professor ("Fatty") Frazer and the Clinical Trials Sub-committee chaired by Professor Bob Hunter, (later Lord Hunter of Newington) were looked after by Dennis Cahal and Dr. John Broadbent, together with Steve Hall, a senior pharmacist. I was responsible for the Adverse Reactions Sub-committee, chaired by Professor Leslie Witts of Oxford and I was supported by another pharmacist, Diana Hine. Earlier in the year, Derrick Dunlop had circulated a letter to all doctors saying "We ask you to report to us promptly details of any untoward condition in a patient that might be the result of drug treatment." This was the start of the "Yellow Card System" that I was to be responsible for developing over the next sixteen years. By the time I arrived in London, a small number of cards had already been filed in cardboard boxes and a small clerical group had been assembled, headed by the appropriately-named Sidney Cardy.

The Secretary to the main committee was Wilfred Turner who was destined for a successful career in the Diplomatic Service. He became the

British High Commissioner for Botswana from 1977 until retiring in 1981. Wilfred was responsible for co-ordinating the drafting of the Medicines Act of 1968. He taught us how to survive in the Civil Service and retain a sense of humour. Nobody, however, had warned us about what was to happen to Dennis Cahal, John Broadbent, and myself one year after we had left "safe" jobs and joined the Service. We were astonished to discover that we had been wrongly advised that we would automatically become established civil servants. We were now told that we would have to re-apply and compete for our own jobs! I had left my secure job in a pleasant part of the country and my share of two privately owned aircraft at the Midland Gliding Club that had been a major interest for several years. I was now apparently faced with the possibility that I might find myself returning to Cheshire in the hope of retrieving my former position. In the event, the interviews were "rigged" so that the people who had run the show for a year were the obvious choice and all three of us became "established." Several senior doctors from the pharmaceutical companies or academia whom we met in the waiting room at the DHSS headquarters at Alexander Flemming House were extremely angry when they found out that they had been subjected to the trauma of a fruitless job application and interview.

The CSD was a voluntary committee whose members were drawn from a wide variety of medical specialities. They were paid only their travelling expenses. The Committee had no legal powers to control the pharmaceutical industry, but in reality it was very powerful. If a company failed to comply with a recommendation, the Minister could make a public announcement that might even include advice to doctors not to prescribe a particular drug. This trump card was never needed because, although entirely voluntary, the drug industry and the Committee treated each other with mutual respect. It made sense for a company to co-operate with the Committee's secretariat and it enabled us to discuss problems on a level playing field without the need for secrecy or the arrogance that bedevils such discussions when lay officials hold most of the trump cards.

The Official Secrets Act is totally inappropriate in the context of public health. I had to breach it several times each day to do my job. The evidence about adverse drug reactions on which decisions had to be made was not secret, having been supplied by doctors reporting to the Committee rather than the Department. In this sense my job was easier than that of my colleagues dealing with the pre-marketing data from animal and human experiments. These data were collected by the drug companies and were classified as "commercial, in confidence." The intellectual rights to data obtained during company-sponsored trials conducted by individuals or institutions under contract to the company usually belong to the company. They may not be revealed outside the licensing authority without the consent of the company. This is something that I have always disagreed with. I believe that all information about the effects of drugs should be available to any bona fide research worker from the first moment that the first dose is taken by a human being. Today the CSD would be said to have been "transparent." Its workings became opaque once the Medicines Act became effective in 1971.

On very rare occasions I had to advise a drug company that the committee had decided that a drug should be removed from the market or that warnings would have to be published. While the CSD was operating on the basis of voluntary co-operation by drug companies, a staff of less than two dozen managed the committee's affairs and processed the submissions of data on new drugs very efficiently for seven years. After 1971 there was a more than tenfold increase in the staff, including many more doctors and pharmacists, a team of lawyers and numerous inspectors.

In these days of word-processors, photocopiers, fax machines, "desk-top publishing" and e-mail, it is interesting to compare the equipment available to us in 1964. Typists used carbon paper and "foolscap" measuring fourteen inches by nine. Committee papers were typed on wax stencils and then duplicated with a hand-cranked "Roneo" machine. Mistakes were corrected by repairing the wax with a red fluid resembling nail varnish and typing over it. To meet deadlines I would often have to pass work that could have been considerably improved if it had not involved retyping. Official files rapidly became a mass of illegible handwritten comments. My statistical calculations were worked with a slide-rule or log-tables and a hand-cranked "Facit" adding machine. After several years, at a cost of £400, I was provided with an electric "calculator" the size of a car radio. The answers appeared when large figures constructed of coiled wire glowed like a miniature electric radiator.

The key document in the reporting system, which is still used today, was a simple reply-paid "yellow card" that was distributed to all general practitioners and hospital doctors. They were asked to record their suspicions that a drug they had prescribed had caused an adverse effect. By the end of 1964 we were receiving about two hundred yellow cards each week. Every one was passed to me, and a number of previously unrecognised problems were detected for the first time. A new drug for the treatment of angina called Cardivix caused an unacceptable number of cases of jaundice, and was rapidly and voluntarily removed from the market. A pain-killing drug called Ponstan caused occasional cases of diarrhoea and bleeding and a warning leaflet was issued by the Committee. Negram, a treatment for urinary infections, occasionally caused rashes when patients were exposed to sunlight (photosensitivity) and a warning letter was sent to the journals. Negram also caused strange alterations to sensation, sometimes resembling hallucinations, starting about half an hour after a dose. They could be quite frightening until the patient was reassured that they were not dangerous. Both these drugs are still available thirty years later. A drug used for arthritis called Thylin that was chemically similar to several other drugs known to damage the bone marrow and cause anaemia was withdrawn from the market when it was reported to have the same effect. All four of these "early warnings" were international "firsts" for the CSD system.

In 1964 I introduced the concept of the "Adverse Reactions Profile." Since we were unable to determine how many patients had been treated with a particular drug or how many of them had developed adverse effects, and because we had no idea how many of the events that must have occurred had been reported, we could not measure the frequency of reactions. We needed some way of highlighting differences in the pattern of reactions when drugs with similar uses were compared. The numbers that were reported varied widely from drug to drug. The trick was to take each type of event in turn and calculate how much it contributed to the total number of reports for that drug. Let us imagine that we wanted to compare two chemically similar drugs used for the same disease. One was a new drug and we had received one hundred reports in the first month of marketing, sixty of which were reports of rashes. The other drug had been prescribed for many months and we had received six hundred reports of which one hundred and twenty were of rashes. Although there were twice as many reports of rash with the second drug, they only accounted for a fifth of the adverse reactions profile for that drug, whereas rashes accounted for nearly two thirds of the reports for the new drug. If we had simply relied on the total numbers of reports we might have believed that the second drug was a more common cause of rashes. This is an over-simplification and merely illustrates that the number of reports by itself cannot be relied upon as a basis for decisions. The adverse reactions profile is expressed by proportions and not numbers. In the above example a closer look at the reports of rashes might have revealed that patients treated with the first drug had an unusual kind of rash, not seen with other drugs used for the same purpose. This happened in real life. We found large numbers of photosensitivity (sunburn-like) reactions to one member of a group of otherwise very similar antidepressant drugs, and exactly the same problem was seen with one of the antibiotics. In both cases, photosensitivity was almost unknown with the other members of the two groups of drugs.

Within a few weeks of settling into my office at Queen Anne's Mansions, I became involved in problems experienced by women using oral contraceptives. Small numbers of women were reported to have developed blood clots in various parts of the body and a few had died. Early in 1965 I set up the first study to produce statistically valid evidence that the pill was probably an occasional cause of fatal thrombosis and, what is more important, I was lucky enough to make the entirely new discovery that the risk of thrombosis was directly related to the dose of one of the two components of the mixture of hormones used in the pill. This was to lead to the world-wide adoption of low dose preparations and to my being called by some, "Father of the Mini-Pill." I was sometimes worried whether the smaller dose really was sufficient to prevent pregnancy. Sir George Godber, the Chief Medical Officer, thought he could detect a small increase in birth-rate nine months after the news was released, and suggested that I might have been the father of rather more than I had bargained for! Some people in the industry, who felt I was rocking the boat, referred to me with less affection as "Bill the Pill."

The introduction of the mini-pill removed most of the risk of thrombosis and, world-wide, benefited tens of thousands of young women who would otherwise have died as an unfortunate effect of what was perhaps the most far-reaching advance in medicine in my generation. I expected and received little credit for these discoveries. Leslie Witts, the Chairman of the Adverse Reactions Sub-Committee, told me one day—"You know Bill, if you don't blow your own trumpet, nobody will blow it for you." More than thirty years after the observation that led to the Mini-Pill and with the knowledge that nobody can claim prior discovery, I shall now tell the story of a particularly turbulent and exciting six years. First, however, I must describe what sort of problem we were dealing with.

The main problem was increased blood clotting, either in the veins or the arteries. Simple superficial phlebitis means nothing more than inflammation of a vein. The skin over an affected vein, most commonly in the leg, becomes hot, red and painful. If a clot or thrombus forms in the vein, the condition is then called thrombophlebitis and it is often possible to feel a tender cord-like thickening under the skin. This is not uncommon after injury to the leg or it may occur spontaneously, especially if the patient has been immobile for too long, for example, on long journeys by car or plane, or after a surgical operation. Most superficial cases clear up spontaneously and are not a direct threat to life. If, however, clotting occurs in one of the large deep veins in the leg or lower body, there is a very real danger that a portion of the clot may break off. The loose clot, now called an embolus, travels up the great veins to the heart and thence to the lung where it may block off the circulation to a portion of the lung. This is known as pulmonary embolism and if the clot is very large it may shut off so much of the blood reaching the lungs that it causes sudden death. This happened to a patient while I was talking to her during my routine ward round at Addenbrooke's several years earlier. She suddenly stopped talking, struggled for breath and died. At post-mortem we found that a huge blood clot straddled the main branches of the pulmonary artery, stopping the circulation of blood to both lungs. Another patient, a nineteen year-old woman, whose diabetes had got out of control and who I was attempting to stabilise as an in-patient, suffered exactly the same fate. She was already dead when I was called to the ward during the night. Such events were dramatic and tragic and were particularly distressing when they involved a previously healthy woman with young children.

The second important group were the patients with clotting in the arteries. These were mostly cases of coronary thrombosis leading to what is called myocardial infarction. If the patient survives the heart attack some of the heart muscle may be permanently destroyed and replaced with scar-tissue. Similarly, clotting in the brain arteries (cerebral thromboembolism) commonly referred to as "stroke" may result in permanent brain damage with loss of speech or paralysis. Patients may die suddenly if a large part of the brain loses its blood supply. Sometimes arterial thrombosis occurs in unusual sites such as the limbs, leading to gangrene, in the vessels of the retina, causing blindness, or in the intestines, leading to the death of a section of bowel.

All these conditions can occur spontaneously in healthy people of any age. Deep vein thrombosis in the legs is particularly common as a complication of operations or in pregnancy. Thrombosis is more common in diabetes and obesity and is many times more likely to attack people who smoke. Smoking was one of the factors that was to make studies of the pill very difficult, because patients usually under-estimate (or fail to admit) how much they smoke. I was amused to read official advice that "smokers should not use the pill." Why not "pill users should give up smoking?" In the mid-sixties, even before the greater dangers of the older brands of oral contraceptives had been recognised, any risks associated with them paled into insignificance in comparison with the huge risks of smoking. The tobacco barons exert a huge toll in "lost years." Nobody can "save a life," only extend it. It is, however, quite easy to reduce life-expectancy very significantly by smoking. It has recently been estimated, for example, that a twenty year-old smoker has only half the chance of reaching seventy as a non-smoker of the same age. Lung cancer, though the most publicised smoking hazard, is less common than heart disease caused or aggravated by smoking. Somehow the combined forces of tobacco advertising and tobacco addiction make people ignore its enormous risks, while the very small risk of thrombosis caused by the pill has concerned every woman who uses it and persuaded many to give it up.

At various times I have come into close contact with four prominent players in the saga of smoking. I was in the same house at school as Sir Patrick Sheehy, Chairman of British-American Tobacco Company. Patrick can fight his corner as one of the "providers" of the weed that I myself indulged in until I decided that the rest of my life was for living. At Cambridge I was an undergraduate at Caius College in the days of the famous statistician and geneticist Sir Ronald Fisher, who rather surprisingly spent the last years of his life challenging the case against smoking. Much later, during my days with the CSD and my involvement in contraceptive research, the statistician Sir Austin ("Tony") Bradford Hill and the epidemiologist Sir Richard Doll became my mentors. Tony was already a member of the CSD when I joined it and I was later responsible for the invitation to Richard Doll to chair the Adverse Reactions Subcommittee in the seventies. Both Tony and Richard had played leading roles in confirming that smoking was an important cause of lung cancer.

Ronald Aylmer Fisher was a Fellow of Caius College. His son Harry was a member of the college in my time and his daughter Rose was on the staff at Addenbrooke's when I was working there ten years later. Fisher became President of the college at the end of his career and died in 1962. A leading mathematician and statistician of his day, he is perhaps better known as a geneticist. I doubt if Fisher ever denied that smoking was probably a cause of lung cancer, but as a "lateral thinker" he spent several of his last years challenging the case against smoking by considering alternative possibilities (the relevance to the oral contraceptive problem should become clear shortly). Fisher suggested that lung cancer might be a cause of smoking! At first sight this seemed preposterous, the fantasy of an ageing pipe-smoker (the pipe was rarely out of his mouth when I knew him). He recognised that lung cancer often follows many years of chronic bronchitis and that this itself might be regarded as a pre-cancerous condition. He proposed that we should consider the possibility that the disability associated with chronic bronchitis might cause sufferers to comfort themselves with tobacco – rather far-fetched, but not entirely illogical. Fisher's second alternative hypothesis cast a longer shadow over the direct-cause hypothesis. He proposed that both smoking and lung cancer might have a common cause. Was it possible that the genetic make-up of some individuals predisposed them to develop both lung cancer and the psychological profile that encouraged smoking? I believe the last thirty years of accumulated epidemiological evidence has proved these alternatives to be wrong and indeed, if he was alive today, he would probably agree. I confess, however, to some niggling doubts about whether we should completely rule out the second alternative as a contributing factor in perhaps a few cases of lung cancer.

I believe the evidence that the pill is a cause of thrombosis is very compelling, but I am equally sure that smoking is a common cause, especially of coronary artery disease. The question is whether individuals who smoke are also more likely to use oral contraceptives. Do both activities reflect life in the "fast track" where stressful jobs and childbearing are often incompatible? In my experience, the risks of smoking have confused (an epidemiologist uses the word "confounded") the case against the pill in almost every study that has ever been published, including my studies of deaths. The reason is quite simple – it is impossible to get an accurate "smoking history" because dead patients can't tell you how much they smoked and living ones lie about it!

That there might be a problem with thrombosis and the pill was recognised earlier in the United States than the United Kingdom. None was more alert to this possibility than one of the principle manufacturers, G. D. Searle & Co., who convened a symposium at the American Medical Association's headquarters in Searle's home town of Chicago on September 10th 1962.[8] It was chaired by the famous heart surgeon,

Michael E. DeBakey of Baylor University in Texas, and one of the speakers was Eleanor Mears, the Medical Secretary of the British Family Planning Association (FPA). The Conference was convened in response to reports of thrombosis in several countries and produced some quaint as well as some important observations. For example, from John Rock, Professor of Gynaecology at Harvard and Director of the Rock Reproductive Study Centre – *"Of course, we in Massachusetts do not recommend any contraceptive method except rhythm."* (my italics). He went on, nevertheless, to discuss his profound interest in the pill! Dr. John Mitchell from Oxford University warned about any study that depended on the patient's memory, observing that "people tend to recall incidents that they have reason to recall." The consensus of the meeting was that there was, as yet, no hard evidence that thrombosis was more common in pill users. Only one of the twenty-seven participants disagreed and one abstained. I was not there, but I strongly suspect that most participants left Chicago with the same doubts about the safety of the pill as they had when they arrived.

In the following account of my personal involvement with oral contraceptives I shall try to describe the events in the order in which they occurred and I will try to keep technical jargon to a minimum. I do not intend to review all the many studies that have been conducted in the United Kingdom or elsewhere and I shall discuss only my own work and publications. Within four months of joining the CSD and by the end of 1964 I had examined twenty-nine reports of venous thrombosis including eleven complicated by pulmonary embolism, all in young women. Two women had died. We had also received reports of four strokes and two cases of myocardial infarction (coronary thrombosis) both reported by the same doctor. Although I suspected that fewer than one in ten of the cases that might have occurred had been reported, I felt this was still a small number among perhaps a quarter of a million women who were believed to be using the pill. At a meeting at the headquarters of the Family Planning Association (FPA) during the first week of March 1965, I shared this limited experience with Sir Theodore Fox, the Chairman of the FPA, Dr. Eleanor Mears, the FPA'a Medical Secretary, Dr. Michael Oliver, an Edinburgh cardiologist who had seen a number of young women who had a heart attack while on the pill, and Edwin Bickerstaff, a neurologist. Michael and Edwin had been involved in the work on cholesterol in my ICI days. Each of them agreed to make enquiries within their own specialities. I described how I had recruited a team of part-time medical officers (PTMOs) who were affectionately referred to as "Derrick's Dolls" (although there were several "guys" in the team). General practitioners sometimes feel professionally isolated and are more likely to give their time to providing detailed information if a charming lady calls on them. Like many busy people, they prefer to talk rather than write; and so it had proved to be. Several GPs had written to say how much they had appreciated a visit from one of the PTMOs and how refreshing it was for someone in a government department to go to such trouble to seek out the information.

The tally of reports rose rapidly and I decided to set aside the large number of reports of minor incidents and concentrate on life-threatening or fatal events. By the time of the FPA meeting we had thirty-eight cases of pulmonary embolism with seven deaths, thirty-one cases of stroke with two deaths, and three reports of coronary thrombosis, all three of them fatal. There was still no scientific proof that the pill was a cause of thrombosis and it was important to recognise that some of the reports described episodes of thrombosis that could be explained by influences other than the pill. This included immobility following operations and medical conditions such as diabetes, cancer, smoking or obesity. Only a minority of women appeared to have no predisposing condition.

During the summer of 1965 I set up the first national study of deaths from thrombosis. I intended to investigate all the deaths that would occur in the following year. My plan was to ask the Registrar General to provide photocopies of the "Death Entries" (which are derived from the information written on death certificates) for all women between the ages of fifteen and forty-four years who would die during 1966 from thrombosis or embolism in any of three sites – lung, brain or heart. I planned to write to each doctor and introduce him to one of Derrick's Dolls and I devised a strategy for gathering information about the extent to which the pill was prescribed in the practices in which a death had occurred.

The work was not without its lighter side. About the middle of 1965 I had a number of phone calls from female doctors requesting a brief "chat" in my office. The first two turned out to be delightfully evasive Irish ladies anxious for details about my work on the pill. They seemed to be looking only for bad news about the pill and when the third enchanting Irish lady sat down, I asked her who had suggested she should get in touch with me. She admitted, as I had suspected, that Monsignor some-one-or-other wanted the "low down" on the pill that he could pass on to the Vatican.

About September 1965 I started to gather information about the frequency of thrombosis in the general population. There were two sources of data. The first was the Hospital In-Patient Enquiry (HIPE) in which the diagnoses of a random sample of patients at the point of discharge from hospital (alive or dead) can be used to provide an estimate for all the hospitals in the country. HIPE is fairly reliable for serious conditions such as a stroke or heart attack that would cause patients to be admitted to hospital rather than treated at home. The second source was the diagnoses recorded on death certificates. With Cynthia Palmer, from the Department's Statistics and Research Section, I attempted to estimate the number of cases of thrombosis that might have been expected among women of child-bearing age before the pill had been introduced so that we could compare it with the number that had actually been reported since. The weakness of this was that we had no reliable figures for the number of women using the pill. However, we were able to gather information from various drug companies and the FPA and we thought that about four hundred thousand women were probably using the pill.

I had seen sixteen reports of death from pulmonary embolism during the twelve-month period up to September 1965. Thirteen would have been expected in a population of four hundred thousand women of child-bearing age. There had been ninety-five reports of non-fatal incidents where fifty-eight would have been expected. There was no appreciable difference between the reported and the expected numbers and it might have been concluded that the pill was not causing thrombosis. This belief was appealing to departmental officials but I warned them it must depend on an assumption that all incidents had been reported. Since it was extremely unlikely that more than perhaps ten or twenty percent of cases had been reported, this was the strongest indication so far that there was a risk of thrombosis with the pill.[9] However, this fell far short of scientific proof.

I decided that it would be worth approaching the College of General Practitioners and, for the second time, the FPA, to see if they could be persuaded to initiate further studies and I arranged a meeting at the College towards the end of June 1965. Sir Theodore Fox represented the FPA and Richard Doll the Medical Research Council (MRC). Donald Acheson, who later founded the Southampton medical school and became the Department's Chief Medical Officer, also attended. A number of general practitioners spoke for the College and its Research Unit. I showed them the limited amount of data available to us and said that, under pressure from the press, the Minister might insist that the Committee should issue a public statement quite soon. Everyone agreed that the evidence was still not strong enough to justify such action, but neither the FPA, the

MRC nor the College representatives seemed to have any ideas at that time about how a forward-looking study might be set up. The College's recording system covered a total population of only about two hundred thousand patients, among whom it might be possible to muster perhaps two thousand pill users. I told Leslie Witts that we were likely to be out on a limb for some time to come. My main concern was that we might be forced to make statements to the public before we had anything meaningful to say. In December 1965 I finished the arrangements for extracting copies of all the death entries for women who would die from January 1st 1966. I continued to fend off press enquiries and successfully avoided any hint that a forward-looking investigation was about to start. It takes strong nerves to have to wait for patients to die before you can do anything about it.

Quite independently of the mortality study, which was based on death certificates and not on the yellow cards already sent to the CSD, I made a discovery that was to have a profound effect on the use of oral contraceptives throughout the world. It would eventually remove most of the risk of thrombosis. Because of the pressure of office work and because we had not been given computer facilities, I had to break the rules and take the yellow cards home each evening with the intention of writing a detailed report for the Committee. Working late into each night, I arranged them in piles on the living room floor according to various characteristics such as the age of the woman, the time she had been taking the pill, which of many types of pill she had used, whether she had died and so on. I compared each of about a dozen variables with every other variable. By this time we had nearly a thousand reports. Over a period of several weeks and at considerable risk to relations with June and the children, I sorted and resorted, counted and recounted the "pack" of a thousand yellow cards more than twenty times, performing analyses that I would now have completed in minutes with a home computer. One evening I found something so glaringly obvious that I wondered why it had taken me so long to recognise it.

I have preserved a scrap of paper recording the results of an independent statistical check on my analysis of one of the sorting operations. It is signed by a colleague, Dr. Max Hollyhock. Like all good discoveries, however, the result was luminously obvious without statistics. This was something that Tony Bradford Hill had taught me. Tony used to send me his comments in copious handwritten notes on the back of old page-proofs of his books (in those days proofs were often printed on continuous rolls of paper rather than loose pages). Unfortunately these "scrolls" recording the wise advice of one of the greatest and nicest scientists I have been fortunate to meet are lost. He said, "You don't need a statistician to point it out; it will be glaringly obvious to you when you first see it"; and so it was. Where you need a statistician most is during the planning stage of studies and when you check your results for howlers before publication.

The next few paragraphs may give the reader more trouble than any others in the book, but I will try to keep the story simple. All the varieties of oral contraceptive then contained a mixture of two types of synthetic female hormone, an oestrogen and a progestogen. It is not necessary to describe the precise functions of each. The many varieties of the pill on sale at that time all contained one or other of only two oestrogens – either mestranol or ethinyloestradiol – that I shall refer to as "ME" or EE," combined with one or other of several different progestogens. Occasionally the product included two types of tablets to be taken at different times during the cycle (known as "Sequential"), one containing an oestrogen and the other a progestogen, but most preparations were known as "Combined" because they contained both types of hormone for simultaneous use.

I separated eighty-eight reports of pulmonary embolism from eight hundred and fifty-four reports of every other variety of suspected reaction except thrombosis – rash, nausea, weight-gain, headache and so on. I then divided them according to which of the two oestrogens had been used. The United Kingdom sales of oral contraceptives containing one or other of the two oestrogens were roughly equal {ME – 52%: EE – 48%}. The reports of all the events other than thrombosis were distributed in exactly the same way, {ME – 441 reports (52%): EE – 413 reports (48%)}. In other words the non-thrombosis reports were distributed precisely as one would have expected if the type of hormone made no difference. The reports of pulmonary embolism, however, were distributed quite differently. Sixty-three of the eighty-eight reports implicated ME (72%) and only twenty-five (28%) EE. There was no reason whatsoever to suspect that doctors would have reported cases of pulmonary embolism in patients who had been taking ME and would not have reported them if they had been taking EE. The odds were less than one in a thousand that the difference in the two groups was due to chance, in other words it was "statistically highly significant." ME was often used in larger doses because it was believed to be a weaker oestrogen than EE, but several people whom I consulted suggested that a chemical difference was more likely than the difference in the doses of EE or ME. It turned out that this was misleading. Although the precise mechanism was still obscure, I had the strongest evidence so far seen that some preparations of the pill were a cause of thrombosis. If ME was implicated in significantly more cases of pulmonary embolism than EE, how else could one account for it?

The health implications and political significance of this work were enormous and I should have been provided with the staff and computer facilities needed to speed up the investigation. I had to continue working at home at night where only my instinct to worry an interesting problem like a terrier kept up the momentum. Fortunately I was not entirely without help. The comparison of ME with EE would not have yielded valid conclusions had I not been provided with the sales estimates, based on samples of doctors prescribing or pharmacy sales, by Norman Taylor, the Managing Director of the market research company, Intercontinental Medical Statistics (IMS).

The Department of Health had no way of estimating oral contraceptive sales. The pill was not prescribed in the normal way on NHS prescription forms; it had to be purchased by the women themselves either on "private" prescriptions or from FPA clinics. IMS had been prepared to do a deal with the Department. They offered to exchange general practice prescription data (normally sold to the drug industry for many thousands of pounds) for access to drug statistics obtained by the NHS from hospitals. The Department had refused to agree to this for reasons never explained, even though the IMS data would have been extremely useful. It could have applied to drugs of any kind and not merely the pill. Norman Taylor gave me the pill data on a personal basis without charge and shares some of the credit for making this discovery possible.

Meanwhile my mortality study had started on schedule and many of the deaths during the first half of 1966 had already been investigated by the PTMOs. Among the women who had died, a significantly larger proportion had used the pill than had living women of similar age registered with the same GP. Since my intention was to follow up all deaths occurring in 1966, and half the unfortunate women who would eventually be included in the study had not yet died, it would be well into 1967 before the results could be published.

It was obviously essential that conclusions about a matter so important to the health of tens of thousands of women should not depend on the results of a single study. Leslie Witts and I therefore made yet another attempt to persuade the College of General Practitioners and the Medical Research Council to set up additional studies, and this time they agreed. It was also agreed that a preliminary report on the results of all the studies would be published simultaneously after an expert panel, co-ordinated by the MRC, had assessed all the available information. In July 1966 the College of General Practitioners started a study of superficial thrombosis of the veins in which sixty GPs took part. In December 1966 the Medical Research Council started a study of women with more serious venous thrombosis who were admitted to hospital. By this time I had already shown that there were relatively more deaths among women who were using the pill and I was only a few weeks short of completing my investigation of the deaths. I estimated from use of the pill by living women of child-bearing age in the practices in which a death had occurred that about one in every seven women of childbearing age was using it. By the end of 1966 there was absolutely no doubt that there was a significant excess of deaths from pulmonary embolism among women using the pill.

It was a disappointment to the MRC and to me, when the College of GPs suddenly decided to ignore their agreement about joint publication and revealed their preliminary results in the College's own journal. Their very small-scale study had been initiated at the request of the CSD and had started much later than ours.[10] Presumably this was a political decision intended to enhance their image as an organisation capable of research. It meant we would have to bring forward the report before the much larger body of information from the Committee's and MRC's two studies was complete. The process of refereeing and publication could take more than six months. Because of the College's action an urgent meeting was called at the MRC in April 1967. The burden of the work of drafting a report on the three studies fell on Richard Doll, Martin Vessey and myself. My study was virtually finished but Martin and Richard's MRC study was still in progress, having started nearly a year later. I had not met Martin before and this was the start of a valuable long-term collaboration and friendship. I invited him to be a co-author of the mortality study that would be published the following year.

When I mentioned to Dennis Cahal that I expected to offer the results of the mortality study to the *British Medical Journal* towards the end of the year, his response was surprising — "over my dead body!" I have never been able to understand his reluctance to encourage members of his scientific staff to publish their work. I would have been perfectly happy to share the authorship with him. Fortunately, however, I was now involved with the MRC team, none of whom was a civil servant. By inviting Martin Vessey to be a co-author of my study and by making use of his expertise on its epidemiological aspects, it was impossible to stop publication of my paper. I disliked out-manoeuvring Dennis in this way but I believe he later understood the advantages of this solution. It proved that scientists working in the Department were capable of producing work that was acceptable for publication. This was rare at the time and I learned that it was to contribute significantly to the credibility of doctors working in the Department. The side-by-side publication of two major papers from the CSD and the MRC in one issue of the *British Medical Journal* in 1968 added considerably to the impact of the conclusions. Sadly Dennis became very ill sometime after this and was moved to another post in the Department, and later died. He was a remarkable man and a skilful leader of our small group. With Wilfred Turner, Dennis had born the brunt of the work of setting up the Committee's secretariat and infrastructure. He tended to play his cards too close to his chest on the "need to know" principle, and this undoubtedly underlay his stress-symptoms during his last year with us.

The joint preliminary report of the working party was published in the *British Medical Journal* on May 6th 1967.[11] The GP study had been a small-scale affair. Only twenty-nine of the sixty doctors who had been recruited to participate had done so and they had succeeded in collecting data on only one hundred and forty-seven patients. Many of the patients had suffered minor superficial thromboses not requiring admission to hospital or causing death. We decided that these results suggested a possible six-fold increase in risk of minor thromboses associated with pregnancy and a three-fold increase associated with the pill.

The MRC up to that time had studied twenty-nine women with thrombosis of the deep veins or pulmonary embolism and thirty-six with conditions other than blood clotting requiring admission to hospital. Although small in numbers, the study was of high quality. Fourteen of the twenty-nine women admitted to hospital (48%) had been on the pill compared with only three (8%) of thirty six living controls.

The mortality study covered a substantial proportion of all the deaths that had occurred in England and Wales in 1966. I had followed up two hundred and forty deaths; one hundred and fifty-nine were from coronary thrombosis, twenty-three from stroke and fifty-eight from pulmonary embolus. One of the problems was to decide how many of the patients would probably have had a thrombosis anyway, even if they had not been taking the pill. With help of the late Dr. Sutcliffe Ruttle ("Cliff"), my assistant at the CSD, Martin and I examined the case-histories to identify any factors, other than the pill, which might have predisposed the woman to thrombosis. To avoid bias, the clinical data had been separated from the record of whether the woman was using the pill so the assessment was "blind." When we compared notes we found that all three of us agreed about almost all the cases. Setting aside patients we thought had predisposing conditions, we based our conclusions on the residual sub-group of women who we regarded as having been healthy before their sudden and unexpected deaths. We calculated that the additional risk of death due to use of the pill for one year was about thirty per million, which was about half the annual risk of death in a road-traffic accident. These rates were similar to the risk of dying from thrombosis while carrying and giving birth to one baby.

This, at first sight favourable, comparison of one thrombosis death during one year on the pill with one death from the same cause during a pregnancy, was welcomed by the manufacturers and by the Department. However, it suited the Department's officials to ignore the inescapable fact that a woman has to get pregnant before she can run any risk of thrombosis due to pregnancy and that there were other means of avoiding pregnancy. A woman in Great Britain is pregnant, on average, for only about two of more than thirty reproductive years. On average, therefore, since she might be using the pill for most of her non-pregnant years, the overall risk of thrombosis due to the pill could be fifteen to twenty times greater than the risk of getting pregnant and then dying from thrombosis as a complication of pregnancy.

At this point I started to be compromised by internal strife over the answers to Parliamentary Questions (PQs). The information passed to Ministers was becoming more and more distorted by layers of officials who seemed to pay scant attention to the opinions of professionals who were employed to advise them. The officials argued that Ministers would be confused by our cautious interpretation of the limited amount of data available. Many days might pass while a draft reply climbed up and down and back up an administrative ladder – Assistant Principal to Principal to Assistant Secretary to Under Secretary to parliamentary draftsman, lawyers and so on – and then be shown to me a few hours before the answer was due with a terse, "Do you agree?" or sometimes, after a phone call, a note in the file – "Dr. Inman agrees." When I did not agree, my opinion often went unrecorded. This routine provided the administrators with the defence that they had consulted the experts. I was especially angry about their attitude to the pill study because I had completed it virtually without support from the Department and against overt opposition from some quarters and because nobody else was professionally responsible for it.

The most difficult were the "Principals," often arts graduates in their twenties, who revelled in their role as amateur scientists and phrased the draft answers the way they thought the Minister would like to hear them. They tried to convince me that most ministers were simple people who would not understand all the sophisticated caveats that a professional wished to include in a statement, such as – we do not yet have enough data to reach a firm conclusion! If the officials did not like my initial response to a technical question about the pill, they sometimes waited a day or so and then approached another doctor claiming that they could not find me because I had been in a meeting all day. An uninvolved colleague's response would often not have been based on the latest available information, only on what he might have learned at meetings days or even weeks earlier. Their advice to wait until they could get the up-to-date story would be ignored.

There was no reason why the scientific advisers could not be more directly involved in ministerial briefings and at an earlier stage, particularly in a matter as important as the safety of the pill. On the relatively few occasions that I did attend meetings with the Minister, the scientific advisors were usually placed at the end of a long table far from the great man, while nubile political researchers, press secretaries and assorted sycophants monopolised the conversation. Gradually it dawned on me that the lay administrators' careers depended on their being seen to be "on the ball." They could not afford to allow the spotlight to fall on the technical person whose opinion might conflict with their perception of the social and political consequences of his results. The earliest pill investigations were among the most important and politically sensitive undertaken within the Department, yet the one person who had done the work from start to finish was pushed aside while the administrators manipulated the data. The myth that the pill was safer than pregnancy "took off" and there was no way of stopping it.

In the BBC comedy series "Yes Minister," there is an exchange between the Minister (the late Paul Eddington) and Sir Humphrey (Nigel Hawthorne), to the effect that "the time to start believing that something is true is when it is officially denied for the first time." On June 15th, about six weeks after publication of the MRC report, a revealing exchange took place in the House of Lords between Baroness Summerskill, who was a doctor, and Lord Beswick, who was not. Lord Beswick, representing the Department, could easily have been properly briefed about the risks of the pill and pregnancy. He floundered for about five hundred words of *Hansard* and was then pulled up short by Baroness Summerskill.

Baroness Summerskill:

"My Lords, I realise that my Noble Friend is a little out of his depth in this matter, but I am afraid that he has been misinformed. I am being kind to my noble Friend. I noted that he was rather hesitant; that is why I dared to say this.

Lord Beswick:

My Lords, may I readily confess to my Noble Friend that, so far as the practice of taking this particular preparation is concerned, I am completely out of my depth.

Baroness Summerskill:

My Lords, may I just repeat the question . . . that of women and childbirth? Surely my Noble Friend will agree with me that there is no analogy between childbirth and contraception, because a woman may be pregnant for only 18 months of her life, but she may be taking contraceptives for 30 years of her life.

Lord Beswick:

My Lords, what my Noble Friend has said about the long-term effects of this preparation is, I think, absolutely unchallengeable."

The Baroness had obviously read her *British Medical Journal* and interpreted it correctly when comparing the risks of the pill with those of childbirth, and Lord Beswick had not had the simple advice I could have given him in a ten-minute briefing. The notion that the pill was safer than childbirth, however, was already entrenched in the minds of the administrators.

Early in July I spotted another clue. Eight of ten patients in my study who had died after giving birth had used a synthetic oestrogen called stilboesterol to dry up their milk. Here was another piece of the jigsaw.

Twelve months passed comparatively peacefully while Martin and I tidied up our results and submitted two papers for publication. On Saturday, April 27th 1968 they were published side-by-side in the *British Medical Journal*.[12,13] The CSD paper now contained even more data that I had been able to add since the MRC report of the previous year had been published. I had collected information about the use of the pill by a thousand living women. This made it possible to estimate the proportion of pill users that would be expected among each of the various groups of patients who died, taking their age and number of children into consideration. The calculations showed that a woman was about eight times more likely to die from thrombosis if she was using the pill, the overall risk being twenty-two per million women under the age of thirty-four and forty-five per million in older women. To emphasise the greater long-term risk of the pill compared with two or three pregnancies in a reproductive lifetime it was concluded:

"On balance, it seems reasonable to conclude that the risk of death from pulmonary embolism during one year's treatment with oral contraceptives is of the same order as the comparable risk of bearing one child. In assessing the risks, however, it is important to remember that women in the United Kingdom give birth, on average, to only two or three children in their lifetime, that other methods of contraception are reasonably effective, and that birth control may be practised during most of a woman's child-bearing years."

In the companion paper describing the results of their study of hospital admissions, mostly of patients who had survived, Martin Vessey and Richard Doll reported that twenty-six of fifty-eight women with thrombosis had been using the pill when only five would have been expected to have been using it. They concluded that the overall risk of using the pill was about ten times the "natural" risk. Thus both studies had shown a similar level of risk associated with use of the pill.

Having been committed to the line that the risk of pregnancy was greater than that of the pill, the administrators stuck to it and on Monday morning April 30th 1968, Kenneth Robinson, the Health Minister, was obviously unaware of the *British Medical Journal* publications or what had been said about the risk of death. He said:

"It is not possible in the present state of knowledge to estimate accurately all the risks to health from the use of oral contraceptives, but those risks about which some information is available, including thrombo-embolism, appear to be much less than the total risks associated with pregnancy."

So much for the first study in the world to provide strong evidence of a small but important risk of death associated with the pill. The inaccuracy of Kenneth Robinson's statement had reduced it to the level of propaganda.

In the Upper House on the same day, the discussants were better informed. Baroness Summerskill asked if the Government intended to ban the pill, and Lord Kennet on behalf of the Department replied:

> "My Lords, the warning to which my Noble Friend has referred is, I take it, the article by Dr. Inman of the Committee on Safety of Drugs, and Dr. Vessey of the Medical Research Council, which was published in the *British Medical Journal* of April 27. This and another article in the same issue, reported in greater detail on the link between thrombo-embolism and the use of oral contraceptives, about which a preliminary report was issued last year. The Committee on Safety of Drugs have carefully considered the evidence in the newly published articles and have advised that, in view of the considerable therapeutic as well as social value of oral contraceptives, they do not feel justified in recommending that these preparations should be withdrawn from the market."

The exchanges suggested that both the noble persons had been shown the *British Medical Journal* articles and had grasped their significance very well, contrasting with the Minister's response in the Lower House on the same day. Lord Kennet's briefing had clearly concentrated on the fact that the risk of the pill was very small and that in the CSD's view it certainly did not justify removal from the market. The debate in the Lords was continued on May 9th with more requests from Baroness Summerskill for the pill to be banned. They were fielded quite effectively by Lord Kennet with some light relief provided by Baroness Gaitskell who suggested that, in spite of Edith's gloomy predictions about safety,

"it is conceivable that some women would opt for a short life
and a merry one!"

Twenty years later in 1988, there was public concern that cattle might
transmit a variant of the disease known as Bovine Spongiform
Encephalopathy (BSE) to humans. Sir Donald Acheson, then the Chief
Medical Officer, stated on television in May 1990 that British beef was
"safe to eat" and John Gummer, the agriculture Minister, fed a beef burger
to his young daughter in front of the cameras. After a further eight years
Donald admitted on TV in November 1998 that he had been wrong to
give such advice. He should have phrased his response along the lines
that there was no scientific evidence (at that time) that would justify
avoiding beef. In his evidence to the BSE enquiry he referred to tensions
between the Department of Health and the Ministry of Agriculture,
Fisheries and Food (MAFF) and delays in passing scientific advice
between ministries. I suspect that he fell victim to precisely the same attitudes that I repeatedly encountered and to which I shall refer again later
in this book. It also seems likely that cautionary phrases during his interview were "clipped." Can MAFF be expected to pronounce on the safety
of consumers of meat when any public expression of doubt can bankrupt
farmers? I shall show later how people responsible for drug safety are
under pressure from those who wish to protect jobs in the drug industry.

In May, very sadly from my personal point of view, Leslie Witts
resigned. As an expert in blood diseases he had been invited by the
Medical Research Council to help co-ordinate their work on leukaemia
and felt he should do this for a while, handing over his Adverse Reactions
Sub-Committee to Owen Wade from Birmingham. He also believed very
strongly that, even though they might make themselves available to give
informal advice as consultants, scientists should relinquish chairmanship
of important government committees at the age of seventy.

Having published the mortality study I returned to the work on voluntary reports which by now numbered more than four thousand. There were at least thirty preparations on the market containing various combinations of oestrogen (ME or EE) with a progestogen. I confirmed that, irrespective of whether the pills contained ME or EE, the total dose of the oestrogen component was the important factor and not their chemistry, but I had not yet had time to analyse the data for possible differences due to the progestogens, the other hormones used in the pill. Progestogens might also increase the risk of thrombosis just as oestrogens do. It was even possible that some of them might have a protective effect. From this point the adversarial attitude of administrators started to turn the affair into a farce.

In November 1969 pressure from the press intensified and the new Minister, Richard Crossman, demanded rapid answers. I distributed a "discussion paper" titled "A Preliminary Report on the Relationship between Thromboembolism in Women using Oral Contraceptives and the Dose of Oestrogen Employed." I had by that time sorted four thousand five hundred case-reports into twenty-five different diagnostic groups, entirely by hand and at home. I could find no differences that could be related to the dose of oestrogen for any of the diagnoses other than thromboembolism. I was, however, able to show that a woman using the larger doses of oestrogen was more than three times as likely to suffer a pulmonary embolism, a thrombosis of the deep veins of the leg, a coronary thrombosis or a stroke. But the oestrogen was only one of the two hormones in the pill. The case-reports needed to be further subdivided into smaller groups according to which progestogen had been used. I ended the report:

> "I am concerned about the incompleteness of the work, particularly since the progestogen analysis has yet to be finished. It is too early to draw any firm conclusions."

It was incredible that a body of scientists such as the CSD could be forced to issue a statement that did not make clear that the work was seriously incomplete and that their tentative conclusions could be wrong; but this was about to happen.

At this particular time several committee members and nearly all the experienced people in the Secretariat had been replaced. We had a new Minister who was pressing the civil servants to provide material he could use in attention-seeking, vote-catching, statements in the House of Commons. Professor Eric Scowen had recently taken over the chair of the CSD from Derrick Dunlop who was to head the new Medicines Commission. Owen Wade had taken over the Adverse Reactions Sub-Committee from Leslie Witts. David Mansell-Jones had taken over as Medical Assessor after Dennis Cahal had been declared too sick to continue. Wilfred Turner, who could have been relied on to keep matters under control, had joined the Diplomatic Service. John Broadbent had died suddenly. I was virtually isolated. Although professionally and scientifically responsible for the work that had taken us to an understanding of the thrombosis risks of the pill and largely responsible for persuading the Medical Research Council and the College of GPs to work on it as well, I had upset the administrators by producing findings that did not fit the stories they had given to the previous Minister. They insisted that the CSD should issue a statement about the probable risk of high-oestrogen pills immediately because that was what the Minister was demanding. In spite of my protests that the proposed action, immediately before Christmas, was badly timed and that the essential work on progestogens was incomplete, my advice was brushed aside. The resulting shambles led to demands that the Committee should resign.

It was decided to call the pharmaceutical companies to an urgent meeting at Queen Anne's Mansions. They were to be informed of the results of my study and told to reduce the oestrogen content of their products. I felt strongly that if there was no way of postponing such a meeting until the work was complete, it would be essential to call a press conference and place an official embargo on release of the story so that the Committee would have time to inform the medical profession about the proposed changes. I am sure the press would have honoured such an embargo. Almost all the manufacturers of the pill were overseas companies. I warned the administrators that as soon as any American manufacturer learns of a serious problem with one of their products or is warned of impending government action in any country, it is obliged under US Law to transmit the information immediately to the Food and Drug Administration (FDA). It was also well known that the FDA had a built-in "leak" mechanism that was frequently used as a media safety-valve. I predicted that *The Washington Post* would print the story within forty-eight hours of any meeting with American companies. This would happen long before we could warn doctors in the UK so that they could reassure their patients that the risk, even with the existing pills, was very small and that they should continue to take them until they had time to obtain supplies of the lower-strength preparations. We had no idea how long it would take the manufacturers to prepare adequate supplies of the "mini-pill." All these considerations were ignored and Richard Crossman issued instructions that the Committee should not hold a press conference because he wished to tell the House himself. I was wrong about the timing of the leak. Chapman Pinscher had the story in *The Daily Express* next morning!

The effect of the leak was dramatic. During the week before Christmas women started to telephone their doctors asking whether they should stop the pill immediately or what pill they should start taking. One somehow got through to me and said that she had stopped taking it and had just had intercourse; what should she do? She was quick off the mark because it was only about 4.00 p.m. Doctors complained that the Committee had talked to the press before having the courtesy to offer advice that they could pass on to their patients. To add insult to injury, it was decided to circulate a scruffy cyclostyled piece of yellow A5 paper, purporting to be No.9 in the Committee's regular *Adverse Reactions Series*. It reached doctors several days after the story had broken. There was no time to have it printed in the usual style.

One surprising feature of this affair was the speed with which the drug companies were able to replace the existing high-dose preparations with low-dose preparations. The Searle product Ovulen was replaced by half-strength Ovulen-50 within a few days. There was no way that companies could have had time to manufacture stocks of the new low-dose products and print the appropriate literature if they had not anticipated the Committee's action by several months. It had not been so much a question of what the Committee would say, but when would they say it? There had been no secrets among the various groups of scientists involved in the pill investigations. I had sought advice from a number of colleagues outside the Department and I am sure that the probable outcome of my work had already been discussed with the industry.

I was always curious how the media had got hold of the story even earlier than I had predicted. More than twenty years later I learned the identity of the senior civil servant who had let it slip to a journalist on a train the evening after the fateful committee meeting with the industry. I still chuckle occasionally, because for a long time I was the chief suspect!

Twenty-five years after this debacle, the Committee on Safety of Medicines (CSM) ("The word "Medicines" had replaced "Drugs" in the title because "Drugs" was now used mainly in the context of drug abuse) seem to have succeeded in producing a carbon-copy of the events of Christmas 1969. On this occasion in 1995, three independent studies, none of them conducted by the Department, had suggested that certain recently introduced progestogens were also risk factors in thrombosis. None of these three studies had been conducted by the CSM or the Department. The new evidence suggested that the so-called "Third Generation" pills might expose users to a small additional risk of venous thrombosis. Again unsuspecting doctors were besieged by angry women before they had any inkling which pills were supposed to be the more dangerous. None of the three studies had been published and the principle investigator of one of them, Walter Spitzer, was so angry that he flew instantly from Montreal for a few hours to complain on television about the shoddy treatment of his group. They had devoted five years to the project and had shared their data with the manufacturers and the official bodies on both sides of the Atlantic. Had the risk been serious, all the groups directly involved in the studies would certainly have made it known immediately, without any prompting from the Committee.

The risk was very small. A quarter of a century earlier, we had been concerned about a risk of death in the order of up to forty per million per year depending on the woman's age. At that time half the women were using pills containing a high dose of oestrogen. Had they all been using them, the incidence could have been appreciably higher. The 60's preparations gave way to "Second Generation" oral contraceptives containing only a low dose of oestrogen, or sometimes none at all; these were the mini-pills. The new studies suggested that more recently introduced "Third Generation" pills might produce an excess incidence of two to three per million per year. This risk seemed to be about ten times smaller than the risk we had been dealing with in the sixties, and even that had been very small. More disturbing, however, was that the CSM appeared to have taken no account of the possible protective effect of these new progestogens against fatal heart attacks that had also been suggested by the new work. There have since been demands that the CSM should withdraw the statements altogether. The new results showed that the risk of myocardial infarction was possibly only half as great with the third generation pills as it had been with the second. This may have balanced the risk of a small increase in deaths from pulmonary embolism, especially when we remember that coronary thrombosis is naturally more common than pulmonary embolism. There was no need for the urgency and I suspect that history will reveal a story similar to the one I have described above. It was misjudgement by officials for which the Chairman and members of the CSM had to shoulder the blame. All the officials needed to do was to read the account of the previous fiasco in their own files. Maybe they were too arrogant to believe that anything might be learned from the past sad experiences of their predecessors.

Before completing my work on oestrogen dosage, I decided to contact other European groups who were collecting data in schemes that were similar to our own yellow card system. I flew to Sweden in a January snow storm and was met at the airport by my opposite number at the Swedish Drug Safety Committee, Barbro Westerholm. She folded my wheelchair and heaved it into the back of her Volvo estate and we set off for Uppsala. It was dark and snowing heavily and I was impressed with the speed and skill with which Barbro handled the heavy Volvo on packed snow and ice that would have kept me indoors. After a mile or two I remarked that I could have sworn that there was a baby in the back of the car. "Oh yes" said Barbro, "That's Bjorn. There's rather a lot of skiing gear in the back and I don't suppose he likes your chair on top of his carry-cot!" The following day with Åke Liljestrand, the Chairman of the Swedish Committee, we looked through their data. Analysed according to the dose of oestrogen, it was, as I had expected, almost identical to ours and we agreed to include their data in a joint publication. Next day I flew to Copenhagen for a similar discussion with their chief physician Asger Pedersen and their pharmacist, Mr. Engelund. Their reports were distributed in the same way. Our paper was accepted in spite of its exceptional length and was published on April 25th 1970, filling seven full pages, one of the longest articles ever published by the *British Medical Journal*.[14]

Although I had also been responsible for the first study to provide statistically valid evidence that the pill was a cause of fatal thrombosis, my most important contribution was undoubtedly the discovery of the dose effect. The "Mini Pill" appeared to be equally effective in preventing pregnancy and, as far as could be determined at the time, its introduction largely removed the danger of thrombosis. It is difficult to estimate how many premature deaths of young women were avoided by the introduction of the lower doses. The risk was small and if the use of the pill in the United Kingdom had remained at the 1966 level I would estimate that about two hundred women might have died from its effects. In 1969, however, about one and a half million women in the UK were using it, three times the number at the time I did the study. World-wide, the number could run into tens of thousands.

From 1971 the pace of my work on the pill slackened. With Jim Mann and Margaret Thorogood from Oxford, I published two papers on coronary thrombosis based on a further assessment of one hundred and six older women who died during 1966. This had confirmed a threefold increase in risk in women over the age of forty.[15] In 1979 I published a mortality study of the possible role of the pill in a particular type of brain haemorrhage. This is called subarachnoid haemorrhage where the bleeding is usually from an artery at the base of the brain. The Royal College of General Practitioners had suggested there was a significant increase in women on the pill. In a very small study they found ten affected pill users and only three controls not using the pill. There were a number of technical problems in their study which made interpretation difficult. I used the same well-tried method, employing Derrick's Dolls for the field work, and assembled one hundred and thirty-four fatal cases together with matched living controls. Using this much larger number of cases, I could not confirm that the pill was responsible for this cause of death.[16]

In May I was invited to the U.S. to present a review of the problem of thromboembolism at a conference on "Menopause and Ageing."[17] The conference venue was Hot Springs, Arkansas. For six months before the conference I wondered "Shall I risk it? Surely everybody will have thought of the same thing?" I decided to risk it (you may ask — risk what?). Kenneth Ryan introduced me and I began, with dead-pan face: "Thank you, Professor Ryan. I would like to start by thanking the organisers of this conference on Menopause and Ageing for their invitation to visit this delightful little town of Hot Flushes, Arkansas." The Chairman and several participants doubled up and the general laughter took a full half-minute to subside. It appeared that nobody had seen the irony in the choice of venue for a conference on the menopause — Hot Springs!

In August 1972 the pill and adverse reactions monitoring took June and me round the world with speaking engagements and meetings in San Francisco, Dunedin, Christchurch, Sidney, Canberra and Bangkok. By 1980 I had published seventeen papers on the pill, quite enough for one lifetime.

3 The Silent Epidemic

The continued development of the Yellow Card System and the aftermath of my work on the influence of the oestrogens in the pill absorbed most of my time throughout the late 60's. I also became intensely involved in a massive "epidemic" of sudden deaths of asthmatics, about which more shortly, and I was drawn into a number of peripheral health issues, some of which have recently resurfaced.

I was concerned about the possible consequences of "recycling" water that had been through the kidneys of hundreds of thousands of women taking the pill! It seemed likely that drug products, including the incredibly potent hormones used in the pill, growth promoters fed to cattle, or other agricultural or industrial chemicals might not be removed by sewage treatment and should under no circumstances be discharged into any river water that might be recycled for human or animal consumption. I could foresee cumulative environmental effects including changes in fertility and foetal development. I have been intrigued to read, a quarter of a century later, about falling sperm counts that might be due to oestrogens or to pesticide residues in drinking water.

A visit to Roger William's liver unit on Denmark Hill stimulated me to look into the problem of suicide attempts involving paracetamol. I included an item in one of my monthly reports to the Committee, estimating that there might be two thousand admissions and perhaps two hundred deaths each year from paracetamol poisoning. Many overdoses followed attention-seeking suicidal "gestures" where inadequate or unhappy people tried to attract attention by swallowing large quantities of a drug that was readily available and which they believed to be entirely safe. Roger showed me two bright yellow, nearly naked patients, a young man and a young woman, lying deeply unconscious on adjacent beds in the intensive care unit. The stories were identical. Both had been involved in a family row and had taken overdoses as a gesture without any serious intention to kill themselves. They had felt well for several days and had then gradually drifted into liver failure and coma from which, with the limited technology available then, both were unlikely to recover. Besides the suicide risk, there was a distinct possibility that patients could take several different brands of "Over the Counter" (OTC) painkillers simultaneously, not realising that they contained paracetamol. The Committee on Safety of Drugs (CSD) appeared to be powerless to limit the quantities that could be sold without prescription. The administrators tried to persuade me that the CSD's remit was restricted to the "normal" use of drugs in the officially recommended doses and that accidental overdose or suicide were not to be included. I disagreed strongly. The clinical effects of overdoses tell us a great deal about a drug's potential toxicity even when used in normal doses. I was pleased to see recently that some action along the lines recommended by the Adverse Reactions Sub-Committee thirty years ago are now being considered. They had agreed to several measures that might have made paracetamol safer, for example by limiting the quantity that could be sold in one package, and clear labelling to show that "This product contains paracetamol."

I continued to cope well with my physical problems. I journeyed widely in many countries and learned most of the tricks for travelling unaccompanied with a wheelchair. I was fit, apart from a severe attack of Meniers disease that left me with loud and continuous ringing in the ear (tinnitus) and severe deafness requiring a hearing aid (in my "good" ear).

As a consultant to the World Health Organisation, I flew frequently to Geneva, helping the Director, Bruce Royal, to establish an international drug reaction reporting system that was later located in Sweden. The greatest contribution by WHO was not so much the international early-warning system but the exchange of ideas and the friendships with colleagues from the various countries. Since all the information collected by the WHO Centre was passed to them retrospectively by the individual national centres there was only a slender chance that the WHO centre would identify new problems before some of the centres had been alerted by reports from their own doctors. It may have been difficult for WHO staff to maintain motivation when their chances of a "first" were slim. Through WHO I met all the leaders of government and university centres on six continents. The pioneer work by Hans Halbach, Bruce Royal and Jan Venulet established a "tradition" in international drug safety work that has been continued by John Dunne in Geneva, Margaretha Helling-Borda and Bengt-Erik Wiholm in Sweden, and continued by Ralph Edwards and many others. Although subjected to enormous political and bureaucratic pressures, the WHO team have always managed to retain their individuality and international respect. It is worthy of the highest praise.

Throughout the sixties and early seventies the Committee's yellow-card system repeatedly proved its value. Boots introduced a drug for arthritis called ibufenac which they sold as Dytransin. Initially it was promoted only for hospital use, and within a few weeks hospital reports of jaundice started to arrive on my desk. There was a lull in reporting and then, after the company released ibufenac for prescription by general practitioners, there was a second wave of reports of jaundice. I wrote to John Hall, the Medical Director of Boots, who provided some sales estimates that enabled me to calculate that the incidence might be as high as one in one thousand. This was almost certainly an underestimate, possibly even the tip of an iceberg since it was very unlikely that all cases of jaundice had been reported to us. Boots readily agreed that it was unacceptable and withdrew the drug immediately.

Dytransin was the forerunner of a series of chemically related drugs for painful disorders. Shortly after its removal, Boots introduced ibuprofen, which they sold as Brufen. Because of the chemical similarity to ibufenac, I kept a close watch for many years for any reports of jaundice with Brufen, but no problem of this kind ever arose. A quarter of a century later ibuprofen was released for sale in pharmacies without prescription under the names of Advil, Cuprofen, Hedex, Inoven, Juniven, Librofem, Nurofen, Pacifene, Phor Pain Double Strength (not a spelling mistake!), Proflex, Reclofen and Solpaflex, to name but a few! The experience with Dytransin illustrates the important principle that comparatively minor differences in the chemical structure of drugs can have profound effects on the pattern of toxic effects.

Sometimes the yellow cards provided a timely reminder of known risks. Although recognised for several years before the CSD was set up, fatal blood disorders due to an antibiotic called chloramphenicol were reported at the rate of about one each month. They accounted for about eighty per cent of all the reports of fatal blood disorders with antibiotics even though chloramphenicol had only about a two per cent share of the antibiotic market. It took me little more than ten minutes to draft the warning message that the Committee posted to doctors in January 1967. We recommended that the drug should only be used exceptionally to treat typhoid and certain types of meningitis and never, as had frequently happened, for trivial infections. The company grumbled about the loss of sales but this simple exercise substantially removed the hazard in the United Kingdom. Subsequently, only an occasional cloramphenicol death was reported, typically involving a holidaymaker with a chest or urinary infection who had bought the drug from a Spanish or French chemist's shop and died after returning to England! I wrote to the health authorities in both countries but received no reply. Months later it was pointed out that although the sales of chloramphenicol had virtually ceased, there had been no appreciable reduction in the number of deaths from blood disorders recorded by the Registrar General. This was because a similar number of deaths were now being caused by an increasingly used antibacterial mixture known as co-trimoxazole. One hazard had been replaced by another! It should be noted, however, that the sales of co-trimoxazole vastly exceeded those that had ever been achieved by chloramphenicol and that the risk of an individual treatment was very much smaller.

A remarkably effective sleeping tablet called Mandrax became a problem when patients who habitually took two sleeping-pills before retiring took two Mandrax tablets instead, ignoring the manufacturer's recommendation that the dose should never exceed one tablet. One patient woke after some fifteen hours to find his doctor and family standing at the bedside believing that he was on his death-bed. A nursing sister, who should have known better, took two tablets and then decided to relax in a hot bath before going to bed; she nearly drowned. We also had reports of abuse of the drug by teenagers. Clearly Mandrax was too dangerous and it was voluntarily removed from the market by its manufacturers.

In 1968 I was drawn into a long-standing argument about the use of approved or generic names for drugs. All drugs have an official "approved" name but may be sold under several trade or brand names. To reduce drug costs the Department justifiably encourages doctors to use the approved names when prescribing. When a drug's patent expires, competitors of the original manufacturer often start selling its "generic equivalent" at a fraction of the cost of the original product. Nowadays, many generics are available in pharmacies as "Over-the-Counter" (OTC) products at a cost that is sometimes less than the normal prescription charge. Once a patent has expired and the market is shared by several companies, the original manufacturer gets a much lower return on his earlier investment in research and development. He looks for any advantages that branded products might have. One might be greater safety but there had been only a few cases where a generic product had contained impurities or was less well absorbed, which might make it less effective in a serious disease such as epilepsy or heart failure. In practice there is only a small risk that a generic product will turn out to be significantly less effective or more dangerous than a branded one. A manufacturing defect is probably just as likely with either branded or generic products and all are subjected to stringent safety regulations.

Several general practitioners had asked if there were any medico-legal risks in prescribing generics or what could happen if a branded product was prescribed and the pharmacist had substituted a generic? Would this rob the patient of compensation if there was an accident? I asked the Medical Defence Union for an opinion. Their reply was favourable from the doctor's point of view but not for a pharmacist or a patient. The Senior Assistant Secretary to the Union, replied:

> "The point which you raise is, I think, not one in which the doctor need be concerned about so much as the chemist. If you write out a prescription for a drug by its approved, unbranded name, you have done all that is required of you, provided of course that you write it correctly and order it in the correct dosage. The chemist must accept responsibility for what happens thereafter and if, for example, the drug which he supplies is not that which you ordered and harm is done to the patient, it would be against him that proceedings would be instituted. He no doubt would seek to obtain indemnity from the manufacturer of the drug or join him in the action"

In answer to my question whether the prescription of a generic would reduce the patient's chances of compensation, he replied that if the pharmacist could not identify the manufacturer of any product that harmed the patient he would have to bear the responsibility as its supplier. If the material had been imported it might be difficult for lawyers in this country to obtain compensation. The manufacturer's dilemma is that if the branded product is prescribed he makes more money but is legally liable. The pharmacist would therefore be safer (and richer) if he dispensed the expensive branded product, transferring the risk to the manufacturer. My perception has changed over thirty years. There have, to my knowledge, been few accidents with generic products. Cost has become the major factor in delivering health care. Later I shall have more to say about the potential dangers of imitative new products which are produced in great numbers to replace patent-expired ones. They are more expensive, very few are more effective and all of them have to be regarded as a potential hazard until tested by time.

It is a pleasure to recall some of the members of the adverse reactions team with whom I worked thirty years ago and who made unrivalled contributions to the success of the system. They rarely missed a monthly meeting and had to study a considerable quantity of information that I provided for each discussion. They did this without payment other than travelling expenses and no other rewards were offered or expected. Prof. David Davies of Newcastle created and edited an *Adverse Reactions Bulletin* providing up-to-date information for all doctors. For several years it was mailed together with the *Drug and Therapeutic Bulletin* from the Consumers' Association. He also edited the *Textbook of Adverse Reactions* to which I have contributed chapters on the Committee's work over several editions. Prof. David Price Evans, a physician from Liverpool, worked with me on a paper on the validity of the reports we were receiving. We concluded that, although there was a considerable problem with under-reporting, those reports that we did receive were generally of high quality. Most of them described events that were definitely or probably adverse reactions to the drugs. Later David moved to Riyadh where he became Director of Medicine at the Armed Forces Hospital. Prof. David Finney was a member of the Sub-Committee in 1964 and, at the age of eighty, was still a trustee of the Drug Safety Research Trust when I retired in 1994. His contribution to the science of monitoring will be discussed in a later chapter. Dr. Roy Goulding was the Director of the National Poisons Information Service that had its headquarters at Guy's Hospital. His service was independent though funded by the Department of Health and was run on very similar lines to our adverse reactions group. It would have been far better to have established the two systems under one non-governmental roof, since the methods for collecting information and assessing reports of adverse events were very similar and would have been less vulnerable to bureaucracy and political interference. Dr. Ekkehard ("Eke") Kuenssberg was an Edinburgh GP and a powerful and impressive man to have on any committee. In 1970 he fell out with the bureaucrats because of his constant attacks on them for failing to provide adequate facilities. It was a sad loss when he was not re-appointed when the CSD was reorganised. Bill Mushin was Professor of Anaesthetics in Cardiff, and we worked together on a controversial issue that I shall describe later. Professor Jim Crookes from Aberdeen and I were consultants to the WHO in Geneva where we put much effort into setting up the international monitoring centre. I worked with four chairmen over the years: Lesley Witts, Owen Wade, Sir Richard Doll and Bill Cranston. I have referred to Lesley Witts' crucial role already. Owen Wade was Professor of Therapeutics in Belfast and later in Birmingham and had published extensively on drug reactions. Richard Doll is a distinguished epidemiologist from Oxford (see Chapter 2). Finally, Bill Cranston was Professor of Medicine at St. Thomas's Hospital Medical School and was the Chairman when I left in 1980.

During the 60's there was a "silent epidemic" amounting to more than three thousand sudden deaths. In striking contrast to the small numbers of deaths of women using the pill, it excited almost no publicity. The immediate cause of these deaths was asthma, but suspicion fell on the pressurised aerosol inhalers containing adrenaline-like substances that had been introduced at the beginning of the decade and had proved to be a rapidly effective treatment. Unfortunately several years were to pass before the full extent of the problem emerged.

During an attack of asthma, irrespective of its cause, the muscles in the walls of the smaller air-passages of the lungs constrict, reducing the size of these passages. The mucus that normally protects the air passages becomes sticky and difficult to cough up and the constriction and blockage by mucus reduces the amount of oxygen that can be absorbed by the lungs and allows carbon dioxide to accumulate. Death may follow by asphyxiation or because the heart cannot cope with the extra work involved in trying to maintain an adequate supply of oxygen to the brain. There are several causes of asthma attacks. Some are due to allergy or sensitivity to substances such as cat fur or pollen, some are brought on by stress, others by chest infections. More than one factor may play a part simultaneously. Asthma is frightening and fear itself may aggravate an attack, whatever its cause. The drug most commonly delivered by the new anti-asthma aerosols marketed in the sixties was isoprenaline. In common with other similar adrenaline-like drugs it works by relieving the muscular spasm that constricts the air-passages during an attack. Before the new pressurised aerosol inhalers were marketed, many patients had used nebulisers. These worked like a scent spray and had to be pumped by a rubber bulb. The new pocket inhalers introduced by the Riker Company in 1961 were more compact, contained a liquid propellant and were operated by a valve that delivered one measured dose of isoprenaline each time the valve was pressed.

In 1964 one of my former chiefs at Addenbrooke's, the late Martin Greenberg, suggested to me that over-use of pressurised aerosols might be dangerous. He had seen several sudden and completely unexpected deaths of young asthmatics who had apparently used pressurised inhalers excessively. I tried to persuade Martin to publish his observations immediately because I knew the Committee would not issue a public warning without stronger evidence. Martin, very reasonably, was hesitant to cast a shadow over a very effective medicine that he had been one of the first to use. Although others might claim prior discovery, there is absolutely no doubt that he was the first by many months to warn of the potential hazard. Unselfishly, he shared the information with the Committee rather than, as many would have done, rush into print to claim the credit. Several months later we saw a report of three deaths in Australia and a warning from the Australian Minister of Health. Martin then agreed to send a letter to the *Lancet*. It was not published until August 28th 1965, by which time he had recorded eight deaths.[18] Throughout 1966 I only saw three yellow cards reporting deaths in which over-use of aerosols had been suspected. A small number of journal letters reported suspicions but it was still not clear if any of these deaths had really been due to the inhalers.

On March 4th, 1967, Martin Greenberg and his colleague, Arnold Pines, wrote in the *British Medical Journal* that they suspected that "patients with asthma were killing themselves by excessive use of metered aerosols.'[19] On March 25th Richard Doll and Frank Spizer from Oxford and Peter Heaf and Leonard Strang from London, using the statistics published by the Registrar General, reported that there had been a forty-two per cent increase in the overall death-rate between 1959 and 1964 and that in the most seriously affected group, children aged five to fourteen, the increase was three hundred and thirty percent! It was obviously going to be important to follow up the deaths and I loaned one of our most experienced field workers, Dr. Muriel Waters, to the Medical

Research Council. She started to interview the families and the general practitioners who had reported the deaths of young patients. In my own correspondence with doctors I learned about further cases. One, for example, was the story of a youth who was a good rugby football player. A friend kept his "Medihaler" by the touch line and if he became breathless he would run over for a few puffs. He died during a school match. There was something odd about many of the reports and it seemed to me that we might not be dealing with a simple matter of drug toxicity. Many of the reports suggested that the deaths had occurred in patients who were no longer getting relief from their inhaler although it had worked well for them previously. Did they need other forms of treatment urgently?

In June 1967 we decided to issue a "low-key" warning, emphasising the great value of aerosols in the treatment of asthma but advising patients or parents to call their doctor if they failed to achieve the relief that they usually experienced.

In my September report to the Committee I noted that we now had reports of twenty-three unexpected deaths. Our main source of information, however, was the annual statistics compiled from death certificates by the Registrar General. Unfortunately these were always up to two years out of date by the time they were published. Although the diagnosis written on a death certificate may not always accurately describe the real cause of death, the national vital statistics are one of the most useful tools available to epidemiologists. In 1967 we undoubtedly had an "epidemic" on our hands, but we might have to wait two years to find out how big it had been! We would also have to wait up to two years to see if the Committee's warning and the publicity it had generated in the medical (but not the popular) press had been effective. This delay was not acceptable; somehow the process of notification and assessment had to be speeded up.

Dr. Josephine Weatherall, a senior medical statistician at the Registrar General's Office, arranged for the 1968 mortality data to be released to the Committee in 1969, a year before the normal publication date. Together with the data for previous years it was now possible to chart the annual deaths in the various age groups and correlate them with the sales of aerosols. Dr. Abe Adelstein, the chief medical statistician of the Registrar General's office, and I published a paper in *The Lancet* titled the "Rise and Fall of Asthma Mortality."[20] One might have expected it to make spectacular copy for the popular press, but they either ignored it or missed it. In striking contrast with the publicity surrounding the pill, the deaths of several thousand asthmatics, many of them children, raised barely a ripple.

We were able to show that the tide had indeed turned soon after the Committee's warning in June 1967. Among people under the age of thirty-five, deaths from asthma in England and Wales prior to the introduction of aerosols had averaged about one hundred and fifty per year. In 1966 it had risen to four hundred and fifty-one, a threefold increase. In 1967 there was a modest fall to three hundred and seventy-three, all the reduction being in the second half of the year after the Committee's report had been published and then, in 1968, it fell to two hundred and sixty-one. We compared the changes in death rate with the estimates of prescriptions and showed that the rise and fall in the death rate mirrored the graph for sales of pressurised aerosols. The steepest rise in sales had been in the period 1961 to 1965, at which point, coinciding with Martin Greenberg's letter, both curves started to flatten and then to fall after the Committee's warning. The most frequently prescribed inhalers contained isoprenaline and were sold in two strengths, but we could find no evidence that the stronger preparations were more dangerous.

In children of four or less there had been no change in death rates. They had not been prescribed aerosols because they were not old enough to be taught how to use them. From the age of five to fourteen there had been about three hundred and twenty extra deaths during the epidemic. "Extra" means over and above the number of deaths that would have been expected in this age group before the epidemic, perhaps thirty or forty each year. Between the ages of fifteen and thirty-four we calculated that there had been an excess of about nine hundred and sixty deaths, and finally in those over thirty-five we estimated the excess to have been about two thousand three hundred! These increases corresponded to about one extra death for every two to three thousand aerosol canisters sold.

I searched the Hospital In-Patient Enquiry (HIPE) data. They provide a reasonably accurate estimate for discharge diagnoses (alive or dead). In 1961 there had been about eight and a half thousand hospitalisations with a diagnosis of asthma. The number rose steadily to nearly fifteen thousand in 1967. What I did not know at that time was that this number was to increase still further even though the death rate was falling. Although many people still believed that the "epidemic" of deaths was most likely to have been the direct result of the toxicity of aerosols, this strongly supported my belief that an important explanation for a major part of the fall in death-rate was a greater understanding of the serious nature of an asthma attack. This resulted in earlier admission to hospital and more effective resuscitation. Although it was possible that some deaths were due to isoprenaline overdose, it seemed more likely that the majority were due to over-reliance on a form of treatment that was normally very effective. It was easy to picture an anxious parent telephoning a doctor during the night to say that a child was having a bad attack of asthma. The doctor would reply that there was really nothing more that could be done apart from using the "puffer." Increasing doses at this stage in the asthma attack would be of no benefit to the child because resistance to the drug's relaxing effect on the bronchial muscles would have developed. The drug itself might not be particularly dangerous, but a "point of no return" would be reached. If the child was not admitted to hospital and resuscitated immediately, it could succumb to a combination of asphyxia and heart failure. In older patients the picture is likely to be complicated by the effects of chronic lung disease, smoking or infection. They too would probably be resistant to isoprenaline but might continue to puff away at their aerosols when they should have been admitted to hospital and given oxygen and antibiotics.

At an Asthma Research Council symposium in 1974, I reviewed no fewer than nine possible explanations for the epidemic.[21] Abe Adelstein and I had already explored the obvious possibility that the fall in deaths might have followed a reduction in the numbers using aerosols or in the amount used during an attack, either of which could have resulted from greater care in prescribing or alternative treatment. We had suggested that both doctors and their patients might have been lulled into a false sense of security by the new and obviously effective treatment. There were two possible explanations for a fatal outcome. The patient might take a fatal overdose or the doctor might fail to recognise how serious the situation was and delay admission to hospital. Several doctors or coroners had used the phrase − "found dead clutching an empty inhaler." Some interpreted this as evidence of overdose, others suggested that the patient might not have died if the inhaler had been full! I felt it was especially significant that the worst affected group were children aged between ten and fourteen. They were old enough to master the technique of self-treatment but not sufficiently mature to recognise its limitations and seek help when needed.

Some people had suggested that there might have been subtle changes in the nature of the disease and that the association with increased use of aerosols might have been coincidental. This was dismissed by most of the experts. If it had been true we would have had to accept an extraordinary second coincidence to explain the subsequent fall in mortality.

Could there be a group of patients who were genetically or psychologically especially vulnerable? Was it possible, for example, that some patients might have an in-built susceptibility to these powerful drugs or were they particularly liable to become dependent on them? Was it possible that by 1967, when eighty percent of asthmatics were using the new aerosols, a vulnerable sub-group had been decimated by the epidemic? Maybe another epidemic could occur several years later when a new population of vulnerable young people had matured to the point where they might be starting some other new treatments. History could repeat itself if doctors and patients forgot the lesson of the epidemic in the Sixties.

At one of the regular meetings of the MRC Asthma Death Committee I suggested that somebody should look at the toxicity of the propellants used in the aerosols. They were known as "CFCs," organic (carbon-based) chemicals containing fluorine and chlorine which were used in many commercial aerosol canisters such as hair or paint sprays, and also as refrigerants. CFCs are now regarded as environmentally unfriendly because of the damage they allegedly cause to the ozone layer in the upper atmosphere. I had found some experimental work in animals that had shown that CFCs can damage the heart, particularly when there is oxygen lack that would occur during an attack of asthma. While I was talking I could see that Colin Dollery from the Postgraduate Medical School at the Hammersmith Hospital seemed restless. He was half out of his seat before Sir Cyril Clarke had called for "any other business." He grabbed his coat and briefcase and almost ran out of the room. In about two weeks he had a paper in *The Lancet* on the concentrations of CFCs in the blood of volunteers! Colin had dashed straight back to Hammersmith and recruited some "volunteers," one of whom was Charles George who I would meet in Southampton as Dean of Medicine some ten years later and who remembered the incident well. The final consensus on this theory was that it was very unlikely that toxic concentrations of CFCs could be reached even with frequent use.

I could find no difference in the risks of death among patients using the strong preparations of isoprenaline compared with the lower strengths. Paul Stolley from Johns Hopkins University in the USA, who was gathering ideas about possible lines of research into the asthma problem, called into my office one day. I suggested that it might be worth obtaining the annual mortality statistics for as many countries as possible together with the sales estimates for both strengths of isoprenaline and other similar drugs, thus reproducing in other countries the work that Abe Adelstein and I had done in the UK. Paul showed that the trends in death rates in Scotland (which had not been included in our survey), and in Ireland, Australia and New Zealand, resembled what we had seen in England and Wales. There had been a doubtful increase in deaths in Japan, Denmark and Sweden but no change in the Federal Republic of Germany, the Netherlands, Belgium or the United States. There were several inconsistencies in the pattern of mortality in comparison with trends in aerosol sales but Paul had the idea that the countries with epidemics had been the ones in which the stronger "forte" preparations were used.[22] The press made much of Paul's emotive sub-title – "Why the United States was Spared an Epidemic of Deaths Due to Asthma." His data were interesting but not convincing. No sales data were available for Scotland or Australia, two of the four countries that suffered "epidemics," so no conclusions could be drawn about them. His hypothesis also depended on the assumption that the natural incidence and severity of asthma was similar in all countries. The sales of aerosols were three times greater in the UK than the USA. The Committee considered that his suggestion that only the stronger "forte" preparations were responsible was an interesting hypothesis but unproved.

Looking back over a quarter of a century and reading the papers again, I am still convinced that, although some deaths might have been directly due to toxicity, the major factor in the so-called "epidemic" of deaths was over-confidence in the new form of treatment combined with failure to appreciate the dangers of asthma and delay in attempts to resuscitate. The lesson that must never be forgotten is that any new treatment must be introduced gradually under close supervision. Drug companies are looking for quick profits, and doctors and patients should be especially cautious when new treatments are massively advertised. I shall have more to say in later chapters about the unscrupulous and irresponsible methods used to promote new drugs, especially those masquerading as post-marketing surveillance (PMS).

Tragically, Martin Greenberg, who had first drawn attention to the problem with aerosols, did not live to see the end of the epidemic. He died suddenly in the snow after completing what he had just described to onlookers as the best ski-run of his life.

The pill and asthma problems had largely subsided by the beginning of the Seventies but more major problems were to follow. One that I shall describe in the next chapter convinced me that the Yellow Card system by itself was not enough to provide the level of protection of the public that we had hoped to achieve when the CSD was set up in 1964.

In 1972, June and I set off on the first of two round-the-world lecture tours. I spoke at a conference in San Francisco and then flew to Dunedin, where we were met by Garth McQueen whom I had known for several years as a consultant to WHO. Garth ran a drug-monitoring scheme very similar to ours. I gave a lecture that was well attended, a radio interview and a press conference, and after a pleasant weekend in Queenstown flew to Christchurch for a meeting of the New Zealand Adverse Reactions Committee. In the evening we had a very comfortable flight to Sydney and the following morning to Canberra where we were met by my opposite number in Australia, Annette Walshe, and I attended a meeting of the Australian Adverse Reactions Committee. As far as I could see, the New

Zealand and Australian authorities tackled drug safety in exactly the same way as we did. Relations with the pharmaceutical industry were cordial but "arm's length" and there were no barriers to free exchange of information.

I spent five days in Sydney attending a conference organised superbly by the International Planned Parenthood Federation. It was somewhat unusual because, although the conference lasted five days, there were only thirty-two speakers, each being given thirty to forty minutes to present their material and a long period for discussion after their presentation. I have been to many conferences in which this number of papers would be compressed into one and a half days. It was an excellent model for organisers of conferences and illustrated a principle that I feel strongly about. Fifteen or twenty-minute contributions do little justice to a speaker who may have travelled half way round the world to present his work. I have accepted invitations to speak for half an hour and prepared accordingly, only to find that my time has been cut to fifteen or twenty minutes because extra speakers have been inserted into the programme. At one conference in Rome where the agreed conference language was English and no translation facilities were provided, the Chairman, who was French, announced that there would be six additional short papers – in French. The audience groaned and when the first speaker started, everybody except the Frenchmen waiting to speak, stood up and walked out! Conference organisers often seem to believe that their success will be judged by the number of distinguished speakers they are able to put into the arena. One way to increase financial sponsorship by the drug industry (who, to their credit, fund many international conferences in medicine), is to invite as many "big names" as possible and then scatter them through the programme as "Session Chairmen" in which role their wisdom and knowledge is largely wasted. International conferences provide an excellent opportunity for young scientists to gain experience in presenting the results of their work and learning the skills of lecturing. To do justice to them in a three or four-day conference may, however, mean that all the speakers are constrained by time. It is better therefore to hold satellite symposia for the less experienced speakers either during or after the main conference. I believe this is preferable to another common practice where minor contributions are displayed as posters in a static exhibition in a nearby room.

4 A Problem Solved, Another Avoided

It is rather remarkable that although "general" anaesthetics were discovered about a hundred and fifty years ago, the mechanism by which they put a person to sleep is still not fully understood. Before their discovery surgeons demonstrated their prowess by the speed, measured in seconds, with which they could drop an amputated leg into the sawdust and patients screamed while teeth were pulled, babies born or wounds cauterised. Surgery was in its infancy until "laughing gas" (nitrous oxide) and then ether and chloroform gave surgeons time to operate with a reasonable chance of a successful outcome. My tonsils and those of my two brothers were removed one morning during the war under "open ether" anaesthesia. A gauze mask was placed over the mouth and nose and ether was dropped onto it. Later, my appendix was removed also under open ether, and I remember to this day how I woke up and asked if the operation was over, only to discover that I was still on the operating table. I was being tidied up after vomiting so impressively that the anaesthetic had to be stopped. Ether could not be used in operations involving electrical apparatus in case the patient or the operating theatre exploded. Chloroform did not explode but sometimes stopped the heart. Intravenous fast-acting barbiturates such as Pentothal, developed just before the Second World War, induced sleep almost instantly, anaesthesia usually being continued with other agents. A volatile liquid known as trichlorethylene, originally used as a cleaning and degreasing agent in the textile industry, was developed as an anaesthetic that was found to be especially useful in midwifery. In the 1950's, while I was with ICI, a Spanish pharmacologist, James Raventos, developed a volatile anaesthetic called halothane, discovered by Charles Suckling. It had most of the desirable characteristics of a general anaesthetic: it was non-explosive and comparatively safe in the hands of inexperienced anaesthetists and recovery from anaesthesia was more pleasant than after other agents. ICI went to enormous lengths to promote halothane and virtually every anaesthetist in the country attended halothane "symposia." Several prominent UK and overseas anaesthetists became the Company's champions of the anaesthetic.

Cases of jaundice following halothane, some of them fatal, were reported almost as soon as I joined the Committee on Safety of Drugs (CSD) in 1964. It soon became clear that the majority of patients who developed jaundice had been anaesthetised on more than one occasion. In the first three years, twenty-eight of the thirty-nine patients reported to have been jaundiced had been anaesthetised with halothane more than once.

One evening I found a vital clue lurking within the collection of casereports that I had taken home because office hours were mainly spent in "administration" and meetings. It was easy to become mesmerised by mere numbers of reports. It was invariably necessary to study the cases individually and follow them up by contacting the reporting doctor for more detailed information. If this was not done, cases would be included that could not have had any connection with the treatment suspected of causing a serious reaction. A case of jaundice, for example, could easily have been caused by a gall-stone or a cancer obstructing the bile-duct rather than exposure to the drug that was initially suspected to be the cause. Unrushed study in the evenings and letters to doctors dictated on my recorder for transcription the following day produced the answer we had been seeking for several years.

By the summer of 1973 we had one hundred and thirty jaundice cases, including sixty-six deaths. In much the same way that I had discovered the effects of higher doses of the birth control pill, another penny dropped. Looking at the number of anaesthetics that had been given to each patient and the date the jaundice started I could see that, as the number of previous exposures increased, the time-interval between the most recent exposure and the onset of jaundice decreased. In cases who had never had halothane before, jaundice developed on average about twelve days after the operation in which it had been used, and there was a very wide and probably random scatter of intervals ranging from one day to several weeks. When jaundice occurred after two exposures, the average interval was only seven days with very little scatter. After three or more exposures the average was only five days. Many of the patients had been exposed to halothane several times within a period of less than a month. This suggested that they had suffered liver damage from the anaesthetic either because they had become sensitised to it by the earlier exposures or because there had been insufficient time for the liver to recover from the previous anaesthetic. Two anaesthetists had become jaundiced after repeated exposure to small quantities of halothane vapour in the operating theatre atmosphere. One of them had to give up his career as an anaesthetist.

I showed these data to the Committee's anaesthetic expert, Bill Mushin, Professor of Anaesthetics in Cardiff, and drafted a paper for the *British Medical Journal* inviting him to be a co-author. He had estimated that perhaps as many as one and a half million halothane anaesthetics were given each year, accounting for about eighty per cent of all general anaesthetics in the United Kingdom. Using Bill's figures I calculated that the reported risk of death from multiple use of halothane might be about seventy deaths for every one million patients in whom it had ever been used or about ten times the risk of death from liver failure due to naturally occurring infectious hepatitis. These estimates were of course based on the number of cases that had been reported, and could not take account of any that had not. If only a tenth of the cases had been reported to the Committee, the real risk of death might have been one hundred times the rate for hepatitis. We were well aware of the risk of damaging the reputation of a valuable anaesthetic and particularly the medico-legal risk to an anaesthetist whose patient developed jaundice. In our summary we wrote:

> "The main result of this analysis is the demonstration that the interval between the last of a series of halothane anaesthetics and the onset of jaundice is significantly shorter than the corresponding interval following a single exposure, suggesting that some form of sensitivity may have been induced in certain patients who had been exposed to this agent previously. Only the anaesthetist is in a position to balance this risk against other possibly more common risks that may attend the use of an alternative to halothane. In planning a series of anaesthetics it may be prudent to reserve halothane for the one operation where its advantages may be greatest, but only if the alternative agents are as safe and effective as halothane has proved to be." [23]

In other words, save it for the "big one" and use some other form of anaesthesia for preliminary investigations when an anaesthetic is necessary. Examples would include minor diagnostic procedures such as biopsies or painful wound dressings.

It is difficult to see how we could have been more circumspect. Although the article had been submitted for publication in April 1973, there were enormous delays in the so-called peer-review process.

Presumably the editor had sent the paper for review to leading anaesthetists who strongly disagreed with our conclusions. The paper did not finally appear until the 5th January 1974, almost ten months after submission.

Sir Eric Scowen, the Chairman of the CSM, and Sir George Godber, the Chief Medical Officer, had discussed whether the CSM should publish a letter endorsing our findings, timed to coincide with the publication of our paper. They decided against it. This was obviously the best decision because it would permit the new findings to be shared with anaesthetists without raising the alarm that would be caused by an official announcement. As the time for publication approached, however, the administrators decided to reverse this decision. They felt it would give too little credit to the Department and would focus too much attention on myself and Bill Mushin. A letter was distributed to all doctors a day or so before our paper. Predictably, it proved to be disastrous to relations between the Committee and the anaesthetists. The Committee's letter stressed that they were "aware of the valuable role of halothane" but went on to suggest that "halothane should not be regarded as the agent of first choice for minor surgery and that it should never be employed more than once within a month." There was a huge difference between an opinion from Bill Mushin and myself in a scientific article and a statement that carried the full weight of the Committee.

During the weeks following publication of our paper, thirteen critical letters from anaesthetists were published in the *British Medical Journal* and a few in other journals. The one I enjoyed most suggested that it surely was time that "Dr. Inman and Dr. Mushin sought a less demanding occupation." Professor Jimmy Payne, an old friend from my days with ICI, wrote in his capacity as Chairman of the Association of Professors of Anaesthetics complaining that the letter from the CSM was "needlessly alarming" and that it put anaesthetists, especially those in training posts, in difficulties because of the medico-legal implications. He felt that the CSM should have given more thought to the consequences of their letter (they had not wanted to send it). The CSM's letter removed the element of judgement that the anaesthetist could apply in individual circumstances and turned the use of halothane into a "wilful act without regard for the patient's safety." His letter, and a similar one from Professor R.A. Millar from Glasgow on behalf of the Anaesthetic Research Society, urged the Committee to withdraw their statement. The response from the profession was exactly what Bill Mushin and I and Eric Scowen and the Chief Medical Officer had predicted and had been so eager to avoid.

None of our critics remarked on the fact that the reports to the Committee were probably only the tip of an iceberg, since anaesthetists who did not believe that halothane could cause jaundice would not have reported any cases. We learned that one hundred and seventy-five cases had accumulated at the London Hospital but none of them had been reported to the Committee. This number, collected in one centre, exceeded the one hundred and thirty the Committee had collected from the whole of the UK up to the time the statement was issued and it suggested that there was indeed a large element of under-reporting.

Unlike the public furore that followed the publication of papers on the pill, the halothane story greatly displeased anaesthetists but caused comparatively little reaction in the press. Halothane jaundice carried a relatively high mortality but when halothane was used in the way the CSM recommended it had several advantages. It was easy to administer, and several of the anaesthetists who had criticised the CSD pointed out that it was especially safe in the hands of inexperienced anaesthetists. It is still in use twenty years later. The same lack of publicity followed the "epidemic" of asthma deaths described in the last chapter when, in spite of our observation that more than three thousand patients had died, there had been no public alarm whatsoever. On that occasion the media response had been limited to two column-inches on the second page of one of the tabloids!

In May 1976 the London Hospital group, who had always been critical of our work, published their results in the *British Medical Journal.* Submerged in a massive paper was a somewhat reluctant vindication of our work. "Analysis of our classified cases of UHFH, however, now supports the findings of Inman and Mushin"[24]. UHFH was their acronym for Unexplained Hepatitis Following Halothane.

I continued to be astonished at the capacity of officials to repeat the same mistakes, especially in their handling of the media. A politician may be Minister of Health one day and Minister of Transport or Chancellor of the Exchequer the next and is totally dependent on officials. Professional civil servants are supposed to help ministers avoid inconsistencies, but must be prepared to change their advice as more up-to-date information becomes available. The officials themselves change jobs frequently. As each of them is moved to a new post, he or she is pitched in at the deep end and often has no time for even a brief inspection of the files to determine how problems were handled previously and what mistakes were made.

When drafting replies for the Minister to answer parliamentary questions (PQs), a frequently recurring problem stems from difficulty with phrases such as "there is no evidence" (e.g. of a hazard). There is no ready formula for explaining to the public that data that meet the criteria required for proof of a cause-and-effect relationship between a drug and an adverse reaction are simply not available. A newspaper report of an alleged occurrence is not evidence. A case-report in a medical journal is anecdotal evidence, and if repeated by other doctors may begin to point to a problem, especially if the event described is one that is normally very unusual. MPs, who ought to know better, may base parliamentary questions on stories they have read in a newspaper without first seeking a professional opinion about its likely authenticity. Edwina Currie was forced to resign as a Minister when she let slip a statement that most chicken-producing installations were contaminated with salmonella. It was almost certainly true but this did not mean that consumers would catch virulent typhoid, because no reasonably sane person eats raw chicken. Before a link between human Creutzfeld-Jakob Disease (CJD) and "mad cow disease" was strongly suspected ministers denied that there was any risk from eating beef. One of them fed his young daughter with a beefburger in front of the television cameras.

Litigation from adverse reactions to drugs is comparatively rare in most countries except North America and I have fortunately managed to avoid court appearances in the UK. My experience of US law-suits is limited to two major cases and an important legal wrangle over the rights of US lawyers to gain access to confidential medical records of British patients. In October 1972, Mr. James Baggott, an attorney of Dayton, Ohio, wrote to say that he was representing a patient in an action against two pharmaceutical companies, G.D. Searle and Ortho Pharmaceuticals, and that he wished to take depositions from myself, Richard Doll and Martin Vessey. He proposed to call on me in London in November. His client was a lady of forty-one who had developed thrombosis in the leg while taking a mixture of contraceptive hormones for a gynaecological condition. A surgeon had attempted unsuccessfully to remove the clot and her leg had been amputated at the hip. It seemed that the drug companies were a softer and richer target than the surgeon. I also received a letter from Mr. David Greer, representing G.D. Searle, who wrote to say that "Since your examination and cross-examination will be carried out by lawyers without medical training, it will be necessary for you to produce in connection with your testimony at the deposition the documents relevant to your studies, including all the hospital or medical records which were used in preparation of your statistical studies."

I sought advice from the officials who said that if the evidence the

American lawyers required depended on my published work, I could not expect the Department to support me! On the 24th of October I wrote to Mr. Baggott saying that he would be welcome to make whatever use he liked of my published works but that I could not let him see the original records on which they were based and which would identify the patients and their doctors. A few days later Mr. Baggott sent me a list of eighty-two questions that he proposed to ask when I was under oath. He said that "A published work cannot be introduced into evidence because the other side cannot cross-examine a publication." This was "big trouble." Any disclosure of medical records supplied in confidence by doctors would have been a disaster for further work in drug safety or, indeed, in any surveys involving the use of confidential medical records. If it became known that a voluntary report addressed to the Committee on Safety of Medicines or any information obtained during a follow-up by one of our medical field workers could be produced in a court either in this country or in the United States as part of the evidence in an entirely unconnected case, this would certainly be the end of the Committee's yellow card system. No doctor would ever co-operate again. There was no question that I was going to show the personal records of several thousand cases to Mr. Baggott or Mr. Greer or anybody else.

On November 16th 1972, I was served with a subpoena from Master of the Rolls, Warren. I was ordered to attend before Richard Guttridge at Russell Square on November 23rd. The order ended rather quaintly with the words:

> "NOTICE. If you the within named Dr. WHW Inman neglect to obey this Order you will be liable to process of *execution* (my italics) to compel you to obey."

At this point the Department's officials still appeared to be astonishingly reluctant to support me. They insisted that this was because I had personally conducted my studies on behalf of the Committee and not specifically for the Department. Normally they wished everybody to believe that they controlled the Committee; now it had suddenly become "independent." They also claimed that they could hardly support me if they were unable to do the same for Richard Doll and Martin Vessey who were not civil servants. They did, however, say that they would send an "observer" to the hearing! This, as my father used to say, would be about as much use to me as last-year's bird's nest.

With such a pathetic show of support and with only a week to go before the hearing, I appealed to the Medical Defence Union. A young lawyer, James Watt, from the firm of Hempsons who do much of the legal work for the Union, arrived in my office rubbing his hands. This was exactly the kind of test case the Union had been looking for. He immediately got all three of us off the hook, at least temporarily. He took out "summonses requesting leave to discharge the Court Order and for directions on various points of law" – all over my head, but effective.

This case was exceptionally important for two reasons. Firstly, it was essential that no precedent should be set which would allow lawyers to put pressure on the authors of scientific papers that would restrict their freedom to publish. Secondly, it was essential to preserve the confidentiality of medical records, including reports of suspected adverse reactions. Records that are specific to a particular plaintiff can, quite rightly, be released to legal representatives, provided that this is in the interests of that plaintiff; but it would be quite intolerable if the records of uninvolved patients could be released in the way that had been requested. Allan Beard, our new Under Secretary, who had walked into this tricky situation at the beginning of the month when he first joined the Medicines Division, took immediate and positive action. He informed the "top of the office" that we might have to ask the Secretary of State for authority to claim "Crown Privilege" to protect the case-records that I had collected. He said that it was vital that I should be protected not only because of the general rules of confidentiality but because the information had been passed to me on my personal guarantee of confidentiality. I began to feel that at last someone in the Department had the guts to go to the limit to support me.

Since two separate subpoenas had been delivered by two Masters, it was decided that the outcome of my appeal would be linked with that of the order placed on Richard Doll and Martin Vessey. The case was heard in the High Court before Mr. Justice Cooke on November 28th 1972. "Our side" included both major medical defence organisations and was represented by two barristers, Thomas Bingham Q.C. (now Lord Bingham) and Mr. B. Hargrove, and the plaintiff was represented by Mr. J. Mitchell. Opening the hearing, Mr Cooke explained that the order from the American lawyers demanding the release of certain documents was based on the Foreign Tribunals Evidence Act of 1856. He outlined the damage suffered by the unfortunate lady in Ohio and referred to our refusal to reveal the confidential documents relating to our research. He commented on Mr. Baggott's contention that taking our testimony was the only way that the contents of our publications could be accepted, and said that, while that might be a correct statement of Ohio Law, he found it surprising. The publications were part of the "corpus" of medical expertise, and as such could be referred to by expert witnesses in England, including those who were not the authors of the reports. He said:

> "It does appear to me with the greatest respect that a system which does not permit experts to refer in their expert evidence to the publications of other experts in the same field is a system which puts peculiar difficulties in the way of proof of matters which depend on expert opinion."

He then went on to agree with us that the questions Mr. Baggott intended to ask would require a very time-consuming review of the whole field of research into thrombosis and as such could be regarded as oppressive. He enumerated various principles on which his judgement would be based. International comity demanded that requests from foreign courts should be treated sympathetically so far as the principles of English Law permit. While English Courts oblige a witness to testify to a fact that is in issue, they do not require him to give expert witness against his wishes where he has no connection with the case in question. This is especially true if the giving of such evidence would involve a breach of confidence. He stated that English Courts will not allow the 1856 Act to be used to force discovery against someone who is not a party to the proceedings. This last point was especially relevant because none of us was in any way involved with the case in Ohio. He concluded, "For these reasons I would allow the appeals and set aside the Master's Order."[25]

Mr. Mitchell, for the plaintiff, asked for leave to appeal against this decision which was granted, but a counter-appeal from our side was later accepted by Lord Denning. His ruling confirmed the important principle which enabled doctors in this country to continue to work in drug monitoring and many other branches of research that would otherwise be blocked if medical information could not be exchanged in strict confidence. Subsequent letters to the US have not been answered and I have been unable to discover the outcome of this particular case.

5 A Hole in the Net

Jimmy (later Sir James) Black and I joined ICI Pharmaceuticals at the same time in 1959. Jimmy was five years older than I. He became one of the most successful clinical pharmacologists of all time, earning his Nobel prize for the discovery of two classes of drug that have proved to be landmarks in medicine. The first was a group of drugs known as β-blockers that became "front-line" drugs for the treatment of high blood pressure and were also useful in a variety of other diseases of the heart and nervous system. The second, which he developed after leaving ICI and joining Smith Klein & French (now SmithKlein Beecham) in the early 60's, was a group of drugs called H_2-antagonists that reduce the acidity of the stomach and make operations such as the removal of the stomach for ulcer (gastrectomy) virtually redundant. Unfortunately and completely unpredictably, the third of a long series of β-blockers, marketed some years after Jimmy had left ICI, was to cause the most serious drug accident since thalidomide. Several thousand patients suffered side effects, hundreds of which were serious and some victims died. The disaster was to stimulate a complete reappraisal of the arrangements for monitoring the side-effects of new drugs and ultimately led me to set up the independent national system that I shall describe later. Unfortunately the need for closer surveillance after marketing was exploited by the industry as a means of promoting new products. Unfettered and even encouraged by the Licensing Authority and the Medicines Control Agency (MCA) that

later replaced it, drug companies were able to set up post-marketing studies that were in reality nothing more than cut-throat marketing exercises.
As we shall see later, doctors were paid by drug companies to change
patients' treatment to new drugs without their consent and at some risk.

The first of the ß-blockers, known as Alderlin (pronethalol), named
after the new laboratories at Alderley Park, Cheshire, was dropped
because it was found to produce cancer in rodents. The second, called
Inderal (propranolol) has been a leading treatment for blood pressure and
angina for thirty years. The third, Eraldin (practolol), was marketed in
June 1970 and was thought to be particularly promising because it could
be used safely in patients who had a tendency to asthma. This had been
a limitation to the use of Inderal. During Eraldin's first four years on the
market the CSM received a few reports of rashes, but the number was
small in view of sales estimates suggesting that perhaps as many as one
hundred thousand patients had already used the drug. In April 1972, I
drew ICI's attention to the small number of patients with a more severe
form of rash known as exfoliative dermatitis. This is characterised by
peeling of the skin and ulceration of the mouth and eyes and it can be
fatal. It has been reported as a rare reaction to many drugs and we always
paid particular attention to it. There were also a few reports of the so-
called LE phenomenon, another occasional complication of some drug
treatments with fever and joint pains and characteristic changes in the
blood. LE stands for lupus erythematosus which is one of a group of diseases of the immune system. During an attack of measles, for example,
the body starts to produce antibodies that protect against further attacks
of measles. In LE, however, antibodies are produced that turn on its own
tissues and sometimes damage them so badly that the patient dies.
Rheumatoid arthritis is an example of a naturally occurring disease in
which the body attacks its own cartilage on the moving surfaces of joints.
Most patients with the LE phenomenon produced by drugs recover

spontaneously. Apart from these few reports linked to pracolol, there were no strong "signals"; this seemed to be just another β-blocker with a few marginal advantages over the earlier ones and no particular problems. How wrong I was.

On May 11th 1974, two dermatologists, Dr. Robin Felix and Dr. Francis Ive, wrote a letter to the *British Medical Journal* commenting on the earlier cases of exfoliative dermatitis and reporting that they were seeing unusual numbers of patients with rashes resembling psoriasis.[26] This, of course, is a very common condition not likely to be suspected to be an adverse drug reaction. Less than a week after this letter had appeared, Mr. Peter Wright, an eye surgeon at Moorfield's Hospital, wrote to the CSM to say that he was preparing a paper about a group of patients with rashes that resembled psoriasis but who also complained of dryness of the eyes. In some cases this had caused irreversible scarring of the cornea. Peter Wright called at my office and told me about the eight cases seen in his clinic. On the 8th of June he published a letter in the *British Medical Journal.*[27] Up to that time, Eraldin had been on the market for four years, but I had seen only one report about a patient with conjunctivitis, hardly enough to have stimulated any action when perhaps one hundred thousand patients had already been treated with it.

In a thoroughly responsible way, ICI sent a warning to all doctors. It had an almost explosive effect on the number of reports to the Committee. Within a few days we received ninety reports of eye damage of varying severity ranging from dryness to corneal ulceration and blindness! The number of cases of psoriasis rose from eleven to forty-nine. I also saw four reports of patients with acute bowel obstruction that proved to be due to a condition in which the membrane covering the bowel (peritoneum) becomes grossly thickened and then contracts and causes obstruction that has to be relieved by surgery. This condition is known as sclerosing peritonitis. It was normally so rare that few surgeons would see a single case in a whole professional life-time.

One glaringly obvious conclusion was that the yellow card system had completely failed to give any warning, not because it was a bad system but because general practitioners simply had not recognised the skin and eye symptoms as adverse reactions to Eraldin. It soon became clear that the system for scrutinising drugs before marketing had also failed. We discovered that similar events had been observed during the clinical trials before marketing but had not been picked up during the process of submission or vetting of the licensing applications. Nobody had considered the possibility that late-developing peritoneal damage might have been an adverse reaction to Eraldin. Clearly it would be unrealistic to expect that even the most experienced medical assessor would be sufficiently expert in all the areas of knowledge – clinical pharmacology, pathology, dermatology, ophthalmology, biochemistry, toxicology and many others – that must be applied to each of the wide variety of drugs they may be called upon to examine when processing a licence application. None of the professional secretariat was, for example, a psychiatrist, anaesthetist, paediatrician or obstetrician. This is why large committees that include members from many disciplines are essential and why the specialists must read all the original material submitted by the manufacturer relating to their particular area of expertise. They cannot rely entirely on the summaries prepared by non-specialist medical officials. The Eraldin experience called into question the wisdom of speedy passage of a drug through the process of clinical trial and assessment, so much sought after by the industry and the Medicines Control Agency which has been set the seemingly impossible task of assuring safety and promoting the industry at the same time! Very few drugs are entirely new or prescribed for diseases that cannot be treated with existing products. There is usually little to gain by speed and everything to lose if a too hasty decision is made to issue a licence.

The first symptoms of sclerosing peritonitis were often delayed for two or more years after Eraldin had been started and quite frequently appeared after the patient had stopped taking it. Although it is obviously undesirable to hold up the production and general release of an important new drug for many years, there is always some risk of long-delayed effects and it is essential that recipients are clearly "labelled" and followed up periodically to see if there is an abnormal incidence of any particular disease. Unfortunately, although it was a major objective of the institute I was to found in 1980, routine long-term follow-up over a period of several years has not so far been achieved.

Towards the end of 1974, ICI circulated a second letter to doctors and they believed the coverage had now been adequate. I asked two of my staff, Dr. Roger Vaughan and Dr. Gill Greenberg, to conduct a random postal survey and they found that thirty-nine per cent of general practitioners had read neither of the two letters. Like much of the huge amount of material dropped through doctors' letter-boxes, I suspected that many letters had been "binned" unopened. ICI were anxious that the CSM should not issue a public statement which might irreparably damage Eraldin. The evidence against Eraldin, however, was so strong that in January 1975 the Committee posted a warning leaflet to all doctors and reproduced it in all the leading medical journals. In the meantime I alerted all of our overseas contacts. Later I heard that a complaint had gone to the Chairman that I had been trying to "clobber" ICI's export market to Australasia!

A meeting in my office was attended by doctors representing six manufacturers of β-blockers. Everyone agreed that the Eraldin experience could reflect a "class" effect. This would imply that similar problems might occur with other drugs of the same type. Subsequently we reviewed other β-blocking drugs regularly for several years and although there were a small number of cases of psoriasis and mild dry-eye symptoms, nothing resembling the severe problems that had led to blindness or even death in some of the Eraldin patients was ever found.

It soon became clear that the drug was too dangerous to use and it was withdrawn from the market. ICI arranged a compensation scheme. There was no question of culpable negligence because all the regulations for licensing a new drug had been adhered to. The pathological changes that occurred in humans had not been found in animals so they could not have been predicted during routine laboratory toxicity screening. Except for sclerosing peritonitis, which was extremely rare and which developed only after prolonged treatment, the other side-effects – dry-eye, psoriasis, and deafness (another complication of treatment that was discovered relatively late) – are conditions that doctors would not have been expected to associate with drug treatment. Cases had occurred during clinical trials but their significance had not been appreciated. After ICI announced its compensation scheme, there was another wave of reports to the CSM mostly of cases that had occurred several years earlier. About half of all the reports to the Committee reached us after Eraldin had been withdrawn and most of these were reports of serious ill-effects. Even if no allowance was made for under-reporting or for cases that would have occurred anyhow, the rate was very high. The Eraldin incident clearly demonstrated that it was dangerous to rely on voluntary reporting by the yellow card scheme and I started to plan an entirely new strategy for drug-safety monitoring.

In the wake of Eraldin there was continued concern in the media and in Parliament. I had very helpful meetings with two Labour MPs, Laurie Pavitt and Sid Tierney, and several battles with the administrators over the answers to Parliamentary Questions (PQs) from Jack Ashley. All too often the answers were distorted by the "Doctors on tap but not on top" attitude that I mentioned earlier. Lay officials would spend days circulating PQs or letters to ministers from MPs or members of the public and then seek an opinion from me or one of my staff only a day or so before the answer was due to be delivered. Ten minutes with the Minister could have saved weeks of defensive paper-work and avoid embarrassment to him. Why was it never suggested that a meeting between the writer of the PQ and the technical people working behind the scenes might clear up many misunderstandings? The sight on my desk one day of thirteen PQs from Jack Ashley was daunting. I would have to check our data-base to ensure that the draft answers were accurate and meaningful. I would have to postpone various important jobs for several days, including some which were directly relevant to the questions he was asking. I knew from bitter experience that little of what I said would appear in the final replies. His questions were concise and touched on most of the weaknesses in the reporting system.

I advised that Jack Ashley's campaign was potentially damaging to the Department and that the damage could be limited by completely frank answers. I could not accept the argument that the answers to PQs must always be consistent with previous answers, to reduce the risk of embarrassing "U-turns." The departmental procedure for answering PQs was defensive and allowed little room for correcting wrong impressions. Administrators should be prepared to modify official views as new information accumulates. They repeatedly fell into the trap of quoting figures for the number of adverse reactions reported to the Committee as if they were the same as the number of patients who really had suffered adverse reactions. They ignored repeated warnings that probably as few as one in ten reactions were reported to the Committee.

Jack Ashley asked what steps were being taken to determine the number of patients who had been disabled by Eraldin. I thought we should try to explain that the yellow card system was not designed to answer this kind of question in absolute terms; it was designed to give an early warning in a very simple way but it could never provide reliable estimates for the total number of patients who had been damaged. There were two important reasons for this. Firstly, we had no means of knowing how many doctors had seen an adverse reaction but had failed to report it. Secondly, although the total volume of drug use could be estimated from prescription statistics, the actual number of patients who had used a drug could not. It was not possible, for example, to distinguish the extreme situation where twelve prescriptions had been issued at monthly intervals for one patient over a period of a year from the other extreme where twelve prescriptions had been issued for twelve patients, each of whom had used it for only one month. This is because, to preserve confidentiality, the patients' names were not entered on the computers of the Prescription Pricing Authority (PPA) where they are processed. There was no way that the yellow card scheme alone could provide answers to several of Jack Ashley's questions, but I had already put forward proposals for a new system that might go some way towards answering them, and the Sub-Committee were very much in favour. However, as we shall see in later chapters, there was to be no support from the Licensing Authority.

Jack Ashley asked why the Committee had delayed its warnings about Eraldin. With hindsight my advice to them might have been wrong. With the limited amount of information at the time, it had seemed reasonable to allow ICI to issue the first warning letters to doctors. They should have achieved the desired result without causing the extreme public alarm that a Committee statement would have produced. There was a grave danger that the media might cause patients to panic and stop treatment suddenly. They could die from heart attacks that the treatment was preventing. Why not admit that we had been misled by the company's claims that their ability to communicate rapidly and completely with doctors who were known to be prescribing Eraldin might be better than ours, and explain this in the reply to the PQ?

Next, Jack Ashley asked if the Government intended to establish a "watchdog" to check on inadequacies of drug monitoring. The Committee had itself been set up as a watchdog, but the facilities required to do its job adequately had never been provided. While working for ICI in the early 60's, I had access to one of the country's first computers at Manchester University, but ten years later, when enormous improvements had been made in computing, the CSM had still not been given a computer to run the monitoring system. There were no fax machines or e-mails in those days, only the telephone and the post to keep the Sub-Committee up to date. They met at monthly intervals and their recommendations were debated by the main Committee the following month. Calling an emergency meeting would require busy members, all of whom had clinical and teaching responsibilities, to travel from as far afield as Aberdeen. The process was painfully slow; the "Watchdog" could take several weeks to raise a snarl.

Jack Ashley asked what steps we proposed to ensure that patients were more closely involved in checking adverse reactions. This question touched on whether patients should report reactions themselves. It is difficult to answer. Their best hope depends on close observation by their doctors and complete reporting of suspected reactions. It is unlikely that patients would be able to judge what events were drug reactions and it would not be helpful for them to report directly to the Committee in lay terms what their doctor should be doing as part of his professional responsibility. The doctor was in the best position to provide relevant medical history backed by the results of investigations. Recently this question has been reactivated. While not totally opposed to the idea, I believe it could cause confusion and it could certainly upset relations between patients and their doctors if the Committee's medical staff started to investigate the report without first contacting the doctor. There are, of course, a number of situations in which patients become extremely knowledgeable about their condition and manage their own treatment. A good example is the control of diabetes with insulin.

Another question was what could be done about reactions that started after the patient had stopped taking the drug? We knew that most of the reactions to Eraldin were mild or only moderately severe and almost always reversible. The only ones likely to become a serious problem long after the drug had been stopped were sclerosing peritonitis and corneal scarring. In the former condition the initial damage was done during treatment and was often symptomless until life-threatening bowel obstruction developed. At the time we were unsure whether this would be months or even years later.

Jack Ashley asked about the possibility of an independent enquiry into the Eraldin accident. I would have had no fears about the outcome of such an enquiry although it would require time and resources and might divert us from work designed to plug the very gap in our defences that Eraldin had uncovered. In the end, by the time the officials had "processed" Jack Ashley's PQs, little of what I had to say found its way into the answers. When I met him twenty years later to discuss a problem about which we were in full accord, he was under the impression that we had been on opposite sides of the fence!

My thoughts were increasingly focused on the difficulties of attempting to conduct research while working within the Civil Service. In the first five years I had developed yellow card reporting almost as far as it has ever been developed, being hampered mainly by the Department's failure to provide computer facilities and staff. Recently some gloss has been added to monitoring with yellow cards by the development of an Adverse Drug Reactions On-line Information Tracking (ADROIT) system. This has speeded the retrieval of information, but the fundamental weaknesses remain. The number of reports sent in by doctors each year is still about the same as my tiny staff were handling thirty years ago. At best the yellow card scheme is a valuable early-warning system capable of drawing attention to potential problems, but it has never been able to measure the size of these problems. This is because the extent of under-reporting is never known and it is rarely possible to do better than speculate about the number of patients using a drug. Voluntary reporting systems such as the yellow cards have never been an epidemiological tool that can enable drug risks to be measured. Although I had been able to make an important contribution to safer oral contraception and had solved a problem in anaesthesia by finding subtle variations in the pattern of voluntary reports, it was unlikely that many other situations would arise in which it would be possible to conduct investigations with this degree of sophistication. I had spent ten years achieving little that could not have been achieved in the first five with adequate resources. At most meetings of the Adverse Reactions Sub-Committee, Ekke Kuensberg and David Finney and other members made themselves unpopular with the administrators by complaining about the lack of departmental support. This echoed the disappointment and frustration that the medical staff of the secretariat had to live and work with.

Eraldin did have one good effect; it stimulated the Department to go to a contractor for help with software. Before the Eraldin incident, I had done some work with a systems analyst, Bob Wilson, using the Department's ICL machine at Reading. The CSM had very low priority but we were occasionally able to get some time on it during slack periods, mostly at night. Data had to be transported by road and print-out was often returned weeks later. I used to joke that by the time I got a reply to a question I had often forgotten why I had asked it or, more often, had already worked out the answer by hand and moved to the next question. In fact this was no joke, it was often true. Bob and I had flown to Washington to visit the WHO centre set up under the wing of the Food and Drug Administration a few miles south of the city. We were surprised to find their computer located in a basement in a shopping mall! The only lift was located in the store-room of a boutique and I had to have racks of dresses and dress dummies moved out of a narrow corridor to get my wheelchair to the lift. The installation was primitive and untidy with great quantities of computer print-out and paper tape on the floor creating a fire hazard. The next day we moved to the FDA's offices for a demonstration of the WHO system. It was suggested that I should put a question to the computer, and an assistant at a terminal typed in a simple request for the number of eye reactions that had been reported with various drugs. After about three minutes a message came through on her screen, saying there had been a machine failure and the answer would be delivered next day. It was – the printout showed the figure 30 for the number of reports of eye reactions and another for the cost of the request – $25. It was clear that the WHO had nothing better to offer than our own installation in Reading.

After Eraldin, I worked with another systems analyst, Eric Middleton, in collaboration with a small but rapidly expanding software company called Logica to design a computer programme for adverse reactions monitoring. Typical of my difficulties was an infuriating exchange of memoranda with an Under Secretary after Eric and I had produced a specification for the new system. I was told that as soon as the Department had completed its "internal consultations" she would be pleased to sign the contract with Logica to implement the system, but she did not think it would be appropriate to show the document to members of the Committee before it had been approved by the Department. Surely, I suggested, I should at least discuss the report we had prepared with Richard Doll, the Chairman of the Adverse Reactions Sub-Committee, and with David Finney, the Sub-Committee's statistical adviser. I received, in writing, the dusty reply – "when I said internal consultations, I meant internal consultations."

Between 1976 and 1979, my efforts to introduce a complementary system that might offer a reasonable chance of preventing another Eraldin-type of accident, although greeted enthusiastically by the Committee, failed to make any progress within the Department. Using the Eraldin experience as a model, David Skegg, a New Zealander working in Oxford, conducted some pilot studies among general practitioners that suggested that event-monitoring (David Finney's idea that I will describe later) could be conducted effectively in general practice.

When I joined the Department in 1964 I expressed doubts to Derrick Dunlop about the feasibility of trying to serve two masters at the same time. I thought it would be difficult to be loyal to a scientifically independent committee on the one hand and the Minister of the day on the other. My subsequent experience was that it is possible to work as a medically qualified official provided one's remit is limited to assessing other people's work to see if it conforms to technical and legal requirements, and to explain current departmental policy to outsiders. It is virtually impossible, however, to conduct scientific research within a regulatory environment. Although voluntary reporting systems such as the yellow card scheme are only borderline research activities, they would be better managed outside health departments where they would be protected against the stultifying effects of officialdom. Immediately after the CSD had been established as a voluntary system for scrutinising new drug applications and adverse reactions, officials had been busy drafting legislation which would give legal teeth to the "Watchdog." It was known as the Medicines Act of 1968, but did not become effective until September 1971. By the mid-Seventies it was glaringly obvious that the bureaucrats were going to make it difficult for me to provide the kind of service that a committee of experts might reasonably expect. The time to move was rapidly approaching. Before doing so, however, I owed it to the Committee to make one more attempt to design a better system that would fill the hole in the net that Eraldin had fallen through.

Although the yellow cards were useful as an early warning system, inability to estimate the incidence of adverse reactions was a fundamental limitation. Eraldin had shown that if doctors failed to appreciate the significance of events, the detection of a very serious safety problem could be long delayed. There were also a number of other outstanding problem that the Committee had been quite unable to tackle with the limited resources provided. Several major gaps in the defences that were obvious in the Sixties remain to this day. There was no routine method for monitoring materials used in hospitals such as anaesthetics or diagnostic agents used in radiology. As we shall see later there was no reliable method for monitoring vaccines. Drugs available without prescription in pharmacies were not being studied. The possibility that drugs could have long-term effects on serious diseases such as cancer were being studied only sporadically and usually only when an hypothesis about a potential hazard had already been raised, such as the possible delayed effects of oral contraceptives. In the next chapter I shall touch on one of the most surprising deficiencies of all. Forty years after thalidomide there has been no appreciable progress in the United Kingdom in the detection of drug-induced birth defects.

6 A Strange Case in Chattanooga

One may already have begun to wonder if very much does go on behind the safety net! The Committee on Safety of Drugs (CSD) was set up more than thirty years ago as a direct response to the births of dramatically deformed children whose mothers had used thalidomide. However, there is still no reliable system for detecting possible relations between drugs and congenital abnormalities. The yellow card scheme is very unlikely to give early warning of another similar tragedy. The association between a new drug and a particular abnormality would have to be very strong, either because the number of affected babies was so large or the nature of the abnormality so unusual, that it would be glaringly obvious. It would come to public attention through the media long before a significant number of doctors had bothered to fill in yellow cards. A more reliable system might not be easy to set up and would be expensive, but another similar tragedy would be socially and politically devastating.

Between two and three per cent of all babies are born with some degree of abnormality, varying from birthmarks or non-lethal defects such as club-foot or hare-lip to defects incompatible with survival such as the absence of a brain (anencephaly). Fortunately, nature has provided a way of disposing of many embryos with gross defects; they are aborted spontaneously, sometimes before the woman is even aware that she is pregnant. In 1964 nearly eighteen thousand abnormalities were recorded in the United Kingdom, of which about three thousand were in stillbirths.

To determine the effects of factors such as smoking, environmental poisoning or drugs it would be necessary to follow up most or even all babies with serious abnormalities, together with a matched sample of normal births of at least the same size for comparison. The annual costs of such a scheme might be about £5 million, a modest sum in view of the potential benefits. It could easily be raised as a levy on the drug industry. The first requirement would be to establish a confidential central register of the names and addresses of the mothers of all babies with anything more than minor defects, together with details of their family and medical history and the addresses of their general practitioners. Ideally, the doctor or midwife who notified the abnormal birth should also register the name and address of a mother of a normal baby in the same doctor's practice, born at about the same time. This would provide access to notes that could be used as a "control" medical history for each abnormal baby. The control group could be used for a number of purposes other than drug safety work. It could be used, for example, to measure relationships between lower than average birth-weight or intelligence and smoking or alcohol abuse. The register would be linked with an agency that had facilities to identify all drugs prescribed during pregnancy and for interviewing the mothers to establish whether there were other relevant factors such as drugs bought without prescription.

Most of the essential elements for such research already exist but few attempts have ever been made to bring them together. A notification scheme for doctors or midwives to report congenital abnormalities to the local Community Physician (formerly Medical Officer of Health) was started in 1964. There is a central bureau, the Prescription Pricing Authority (PPA), that processes all NHS prescriptions to reimburse pharmacists. There is, or perhaps was until I left the Department in 1980, an arrangement for interviewing doctors to obtain clinical details and information about drug use using a team of about a hundred part-time medical officers ("Derrick's Dolls" referred to in Chapter 2). This team could easily have been expanded. Community nurses or health visitors could be recruited to interview mothers and enquire if there was any previous history of abnormal births in the family, whether they smoked or had used other "recreational" drugs, were exposed to occupational or environmental hazards or had used drugs bought in pharmacies without a prescription. Those involved could obtain the required information about an abnormal birth and a normal "control" birth during the same visit to the practice (as was done in my studies of thrombosis and oral contraceptives).

There is no arrangement for recording exposure to drugs bought "over-the-counter" (OTC). The recent policy of freeing potent drugs from prescription controls is presumably an attempt to reduce NHS costs, a very desirable objective but one that is not without some risk. It is very unlikely that a drug would be released for OTC sale until it had been in widespread use for many years without apparent harm. Good examples of powerful drugs that have been placed on the OTC lists are Tagamet, Zantac, Axid and Pepcid used for treatment of stomach ulcers. They are nowadays freely available to treat indigestion from whatever cause and however trivial (e.g. after a binge). They are highly effective in this role and would not have been released if the authorities had any serious concerns about their safety. However, they could mask the symptoms of a developing cancer leading to delayed diagnosis and treatment. It remains to be seen if the change of policy has set a dangerous precedent. Nearly twenty years ago there was some concern that Tagamet, the first member of the group, might affect the incidence of cancer of the lower bowel. Fortunately this has never been confirmed. However, when I set up the unit in Southampton that I shall describe later, I decided that the identities of seventy-five thousand patients should be stored in the Unit in case we might need to mount a future study, perhaps as late as the early part of the twenty-first century! Cancer may not develop for a quarter of a century after exposure to its cause (e.g. tobacco smoke).

An example of the need to establish a register of drug exposures during pregnancy was a little publicised tragedy caused by stilboesterol, a synthetic sex hormone once used extensively in gynaecology or to dry up the flow of milk in women who wished to feed their babies artificially. It can also be used to suppress testicular function in men with prostate cancer. Stilboesterol was found, as a result of a superb piece of detective work in the US, to have caused an unusual form of cancer of the vagina, but not the vagina of the woman who used it! The cancer attacked teenage girls who had never used stilboesterol themselves but whose mothers had been treated with it while they were pregnant.[28] Teenagers sometimes found themselves starting womanhood after surgical removal of their reproductive organs.

The placenta offers a natural barrier to the passage into the foetus of many, but unfortunately not all, noxious substances. All new drugs now have to pass tests in pregnant animals and this is a major step forwards after thalidomide, but it is not infallible because laboratory animals are not always good predictors of hazards to humans. The human foetal organs are formed and are most sensitive to so-called teratogens (substances that cause congenital defects) during the first six to eight weeks after fertilisation. The timing of exposure is critical; for example, if a mother had caught German measles in the fourth month of pregnancy, it could not have been responsible for a "hole in the heart" because the apertures that connect the various chambers of the heart during its early development would already have closed. However, a fourth-month exposure might cause deafness because the hearing organ is not completely formed until the end of that month. Other factors such as smoking or alcohol may harm the developing child at any stage in pregnancy. As an aside, I was slightly amazed (hardly amused) to hear some years ago of a plea that has apparently been suggested in US courts. It is called the Plea of Wrongful Birth where a child with a severe hereditary or acquired disability that was diagnosable before birth, sues its parents for not having had it aborted! It might be reasonable for a child that has been irreparably damaged by something that its mother did voluntarily during pregnancy, such as smoking or taking alcohol or addictive drugs, to claim for compensation in later life.

Some defects are hereditary, passed on from generation to generation, and are unlikely to have been due to environmental factors or drugs, although it is not impossible that the initial ancestral mutation that started a chain of non-lethal inherited defects could have been an environmental exposure to a toxic substance. I have seen photographs from the Zambezi where there are families who have dramatic "lobster-claw" deformities of the feet and frequently the hands as well. Their feet are split into two halves so that their V-shaped footprints somewhat resemble those of an ostrich. The "Ostrich-Men" are capable of remarkable dexterity such as pouring from a bottle held in one foot to a glass held in the other. Several members of a family may be affected and the condition causes little disability for people who walk barefoot. This is a mutation that can have no immediate link with exposure to a teratogen during the pregnancy of individual mothers in the affected community, but one cannot entirely rule out the possibility that the ancestral mutation, the first ostrich man or woman, was caused by some form of chemical exposure. Closer to home, it seems possible that limb defects in children may have occurred as a result of use of thalidomide by a grandmother. We had anticipated the possibility of second or third generation teratogenicity at the time the CSD first set up the yellow card system. We realised in the early 60's that we were speculating about events that might not be seen until the turn of the century and we still have no scheme that would even identify abnormalities in the first generation.

Another example of an hereditary abnormality is achondroplasia, a condition causing dwarfism, in which the bones of the limbs and some bones in the skull fail to grow to their normal length. This is a fairly common malformation that must be clearly distinguished when studying relationships between drugs and abnormalities. Achondroplasia may occur as a spontaneous mutation in a family that can trace no similar abnormality among any of its ancestors. The abnormality is so characteristic that one can be virtually certain that no environmental factor has been responsible, nor can anything that the mother has taken during pregnancy have caused it. The abnormality is particularly interesting because nothing is missing other than whatever chemical factor it is that switches on the genes that control the length that bones should grow. The defects are always symmetrical, and only the bones are affected. All the organs, including the brain, are normal. I was a student at Cambridge with a dwarf who became prominent in research in restricted growth. He had an even more famous name – Sir William Shakespeare Bt. His achondroplasia was passed to his son Thomas and his granddaughter.

Sorting out hereditary from acquired abnormalities can be extremely complicated because of the incompleteness of historical records. An individual with an hereditary condition can only have inherited it from an ancestor. Aunts and uncles are not ancestors, only two parents, four grandparents and eight great-grandparents and so on, but the presence of the same abnormality in one or more of the siblings or a cousin of an ancestor may provide a clue to a common ancestor with the defect further back in the family history. It is reasonable to assume that a history of a congenital abnormality in any close relative considerably reduces the chances that a drug has been responsible.

If thalidomide was the first large-scale disaster in which the foetus was involved, it was certainly not the first occasion on which the possibility that chemicals might damage the foetus had been considered. Buried among the files I left behind at the Department are some documents describing tests conducted shortly before the second World War by one of the American chemical companies producing refrigerating agents. I came across them while looking into the potential dangers of similar agents used as propellants in asthma inhalers. The offspring of animals that had been kept in an atmosphere containing high concentrations of "CFC" (chlorofluorocarbon) were reported to have been carefully examined and found to be quite normal and it was recorded very clearly that fertility was unaffected (e.g. normal litter-size). It stretches the imagination too far to suppose that drugs had never been considered as possible teratogens by thousands of scientists working in university or drug company laboratories many years before the thalidomide disaster. It is similarly improbable that all the intelligent people who put together the first computers and their software could have failed to understand the consequences of omitting two of the four digits required to characterise a date. The "Millennium Bug" seems to be a typical example of planned obsolescence built into a product by cynical businessmen and programmers who anticipated a need to boost sales and preserve jobs in the future when computers and software became less expensive.

In 1962 the Swedish National Board of Health, sensitised by the thalidomide tragedy, banned a drug called meclozine, because they thought it might be causing abnormalities. Meclozine was sold in the UK under various names such as Ancolan and Ancoloxin, as a treatment for vomiting in pregnancy. In 1964 Dr. Richard Smithells, a Liverpool paediatrician, published a preliminary account of a study of two hundred and nineteen women who had been treated with meclozine during the first twelve weeks of pregnancy. He could not find any hazard.[29] After discussion with Richard, I reviewed the literature from the UK and other countries and tried to make sense of the reports we had received. The assessment was complicated because many pregnant women, whether they subsequently give birth to a normal child or not, suffered from early-morning sickness and took anti-nauseant drugs such as meclozine that could be bought without a prescription. A product appropriately known as Sea-Legs used by holidaymakers also contained meclozine. In my view the literature contained no positive evidence of damage to the human embryo but the data were mostly too poor to reach a firm conclusion one way or the other. The Committee agreed and complained (yet again) about our lack of facilities to investigate this kind of issue.

Fourteen years later in 1978, the number of pregnancies included in Dick Smithells' investigation had grown to nearly two thousand three hundred and again he reported completely negative results.[30] He pointed out that "drug histories" depending on memory are notoriously capricious. There were often serious uncertainties about whether or at what stage in pregnancy a woman had used meclozine. He had a record of the names of doctors and patients and the date prescriptions had been dispensed but this only identified prescribed medicines. He had to rely for some vital information on what the mothers remembered. In spite of these weaknesses, however, his data were the best that could be obtained in Britain. He reported that congenital abnormalities had affected 1.8 per cent of all babies in the survey and that 1.5 per cent of the sub-group who had used meclozine had abnormalities In other words there was no evidence that the drug was a teratogen. No other evidence to the contrary emerged from studies in several countries.

Another problem arose about the same time as the meclozine case and was more difficult to deal with. In the 50's it was not unusual to use a mixture of female sex hormones, very similar to those used for contraception, as a test for pregnancy. The test mixture was taken for two days and if the woman then had a "show" resembling a period, the test was said to have been "negative." If she did not bleed, the test was "positive" and she was assumed to be pregnant. In 1958, three years before McBride published his letter about thalidomide, the geneticist J. H. Edwards had suggested that these tests could provide exactly "the type of insult likely to cause foetal malformations."[31] Few people thought this was likely, but an alert paediatrician, Dr. Isabel Gal of Queen Mary's Hospital for Children in Carshalton, England, had noted Edward's concern and had started a small study in Surrey. She wrote to me in April 1965 asking if she could use the drug classification I had developed for the Committee, which I was happy for her to do.

In May 1967 Dr. Gal and her chief at Carshalton, Dr. Brian Kirman, sent a letter to *Nature* saying that they believed there was an association between hormone pregnancy tests (HPT) and the condition known as spina bifida, where a child is born with a defect of the lower spine that often causes paralysis of the lower limbs. Sometimes there may also be a defect in the brain leading to great enlargement of the child's head (hydrocephalus) which is usually treated by inserting a valve inside the skull to drain away the excess fluid. Dr. Gal had interviewed one hundred mothers whose babies had spina bifida and found that nineteen of them had used HPT. She had then interviewed another one hundred mothers of normal children of whom only four had used HPT.[32]

Although this may have amounted to prima facie evidence of a possible drug effect, there were several technical reasons why the evidence might be flawed. Firstly, the cases had been referred to one hospital from a wide area in the South of England, while the controls were collected locally. GPs often take advice about prescribing from only one or two local consultants or they may be influenced by what they learn at postgraduate refresher courses. I had already seen a fascinating example of how easily reporting of suspected adverse reactions could be influenced in unexpected ways. Several months earlier I had become quite concerned that drugs used to treat epilepsy in a pregnant woman might be associated with hare-lip or cleft-palate. I had noted an imbalance among the reports reaching the CSD. There were many more reports of lip or palate deformities among the children of epileptic women using certain anti-convulsant drugs than among children of non-epileptics. It was possible that the abnormalities were related to the epilepsy rather than its treatment, but the difference I had seen was far larger than could be accounted for in this way. I wrote a note in my monthly report to the Committee which was probably as wide of the mark as I have ever been. Months later I spotted that virtually all the CSD's reports had come from only three or four towns on the south coast of England! Later still I discovered that a young paediatrician, Dr. Sam Meadow, had given a talk to GPs at a post-graduate centre at which he had discussed the possible role of anticon-vulsant drugs. This had stimulated several GPs to report their cases to the CSD. We had hardly any similar reports from anywhere else in the whole of the country.

It seemed distinctly possible that Dr. Gal's observations reflected nothing more than less frequent use of HPT by doctors in her locality and that she had relied on the local experience when comparing use by doctors in the much larger catchment area from which her cases had been collected. Since her survey depended on the mother's memory, one would expect that the mothers of abnormal children might have been more accurate in their replies. Experience of adversity sharpens the memory remarkably when it comes to enquiry about its possible cause. Then there also was a point of fundamental importance confirmed by Professor Sir Norman Jeffcoate, the President of the Royal College of Obstetricians and Gynaecologists, who was one of the Committee's advisers. HPT, he agreed, was far more likely to have been used by women who had previously delivered a deformed child and who would be afraid of bearing another. Finally, and most important of all, the average time of exposure of Dr. Gal's cases was probably about thirty-eight days after conception. The brain and spinal cord develop from an enfolding of cells on the surface of the embryo called the neural tube, a stage in development that is completed about the twenty-eighth day. If the average time of exposure of Dr. Gal's cases was thirty-eight days, this would mean that half of them would have been exposed after thirty-eight days so half of the baby's spines could not have been affected by HPT.

After meeting Dr. Gal and her colleagues and discussing her views with the Committee, I wrote to her to suggest that she should publish them in greater detail than had been possible in the brief note in *Nature*. I thought this would enable the matter to be debated quietly by experts or even possibly disposed of by peer review without publication. I may have misjudged the effect that this advice might have on Dr. Gal and should perhaps have said more about the reasons why we were not enthusiastic about her letter to *Nature*. I was not, however, free to pass on some of the Committee's thoughts and future plans and could not take Dr. Gal completely into my confidence. This constraint was to lead to a great deal of avoidable trouble later and adds further support to the case against establishing drug safety monitoring within the Department of Health. The Committee's view was that HPT was not essential because other methods for diagnosing pregnancy were available; but there was another aspect that had to be absolutely taboo. Most of the hormones that could be used for the pregnancy test also had important applications in the treatment of various gynaecological disturbances. Even more important, the HPT hormones were also very similar to the hormone mixtures used for contraception. A thalidomide-type scare in the media could easily cause panic among women using oral contraceptives. What would happen, for example, if a woman started to take the pill before she was aware that she was already pregnant? On the one hand we had Dr. Gal's suspicion of a possible danger to the foetus and, on the other hand, a very real danger that publicity might cause women to stop using oral contraceptives or other preparations that were important in the treatment of a variety of gynaecological disorders. I was advised not to discuss these possibilities with anybody in case the idea that the HPT problem might have much wider repercussions inadvertently slipped out, though I can hardly believe many people would not have thought of it themselves.

At least twelve different hormone mixtures had been advertised for pregnancy testing. They included Roussel's Amenorrhone Forte, which was identical in composition with Marshall's aptly named Pregornot, and similar to Organon's Menstrogen and Schering's Primodos, the market leader. The complexity of the situation made it very difficult for the Committee to undertake any action that would stop their use as a pregnancy test without compromising their other important uses. We felt that a low-key publication by Dr. Gal could lead to further research, and I advised the Committee not to comment officially at this point. I wish I hadn't.

Our inability to detect teratogenic drug effects, one of several fundamental defects of the CSD's yellow card system, had been obvious since the scheme had set up in 1964. There had been prolonged but unfruitful discussions with the Medical Research Council and other expert bodies. Any contribution by the yellow card scheme depended on the chance that prescribers would not only recognise links between maternal drug use and abnormalities seen several months later and that they would then report them in sufficient numbers to raise suspicions. We decided to design a study that might be the prototype of a national scheme (that still eludes us) mentioned at the beginning of this chapter. In collaboration with the Office of Population Censuses and Surveys (OPCS), Dr. Gill Greenberg and I began a pilot study in 1969. As well as studying HPT to see if we could confirm or refute Dr.Gal's hypothesis, we intended to look into the possibility there might be a link between anti-epileptic drugs and infants with cleft palate, and we wanted to lay the ghost of the suggestion that morning sickness pills might be producing abnormalities. The study was modelled on the one I had done with the pill three years earlier, but it would be necessary to continue it for several years to assemble sufficiently large groups of children with each type of abnormality to allow valid conclusions to be drawn.

Progress with this study was lamentably slow, largely because higher priority had been given to concurrent problems with oral contraceptives, asthma deaths, the Eraldin disaster and the lack of equipment and staff. We were not able to send a letter to the *British Medical Journal* reporting some preliminary results until April 1975.[33] By that time we had examined one hundred and forty-nine pregnancies with a variety of abnormalities together with the same number of normal ones. HPT had been used by twenty-three mothers of abnormal babies compared with only eight of the controls. At first sight it seemed that our preliminary results tended to support those of Dr. Gal. Although we could not rule out this possibility entirely, it seemed much more likely, as Norman Jeffcoate had predicted, that the reason for doing the test, such as the previous birth of an abnormal baby, would eventually prove to be the important factor and not the test itself. A woman who had already born an abnormal child was much more likely to bear another. Although there were more women who had used HPT in the group as a whole, this was not true in the small number of cases of spina bifida it included, so we had added nothing to the case presented eight years earlier by Dr. Gal.

There was no media response to our short paper and so, two months later in June 1975, the Committee finally decided that it was probably safe to recommend that the hormone test was not essential since there were other effective methods for diagnosing pregnancy. The same hormone mixtures were still required for treatment of menstrual disorders. We avoided any reference to the fact that a woman who conceived while taking the pill might think she was at risk of producing an abnormal baby because she had taken the hormones at or near the moment of conception.

Shortly before our letter appeared, The *Sunday Times* printed a well written and largely accurate story by Oliver Gillie. Unfortunately it contributed to a misunderstanding about the reasons why we had started the Committee's study about eight years earlier. Dr. Gal assumed her study had provided the stimulus for ours. However, the inadequacy of voluntary reporting of birth defects had been recognised even before the Committee was established in 1964. Had we been convinced by Dr. Gal's study, the Committee would have banned HPT immediately in 1967; we would not have waited for the results of an investigation which might take several years to complete.

I had hoped that the pace of our study could eventually be increased to include at least two thousand cases and the same number of controls each year. This proved to be hopelessly over-ambitious. Under-funding and under-staffing eventually limited it to a total of eight hundred and thirty-six abnormal babies and the same number of controls, collected over several years.[34] As we had suspected, four times as many mothers of abnormal children than "control" mothers had a family history of previous abnormalities or had themselves borne abnormal children in the past. This was more than enough to account for the small excess of HPT use we had noted in our earlier report. Moreover, the use of HPT was evenly spread among the mothers of babies with a whole range of abnormalities including those that were hereditary that could not be drug-related. There was no suggestion of any specific connection with spina bifida.

Dr. Gal remained unconvinced and perhaps somewhat aggrieved she had not been given more recognition by the Committee and the Department. She had pinned her hopes for future research grants on this work. She sought my help and I wrote to the Medical Research Council, the Department and several manufacturers in support of her applications for funding but without effect. She also enlisted the help of Jack Ashley who pressed for a public enquiry into the safety of HPT. The Minister,

Roland Moyle, was advised against it by his officials. I could not understand the arguments against such an enquiry other than the cost to the taxpayer. At least we would have an opportunity to prepare GPs so they could reassure any women who had started taking oral contraceptives without realising that they were pregnant.

Professor Koller of Mainz, an international authority on congenital abnormality, wrote to me and we met in Germany. He had performed a technically admirable study in nearly eight thousand women, of whom a sub-group of three hundred and thirty-seven had used HPT. This was the kind of study I had dreamed of being able to do myself. If HPT was not a teratogen, Koller would have expected five HPT- exposed children to have been born with a major defect; he found six. He would also have expected about seventy-five children with minor defects such as birthmarks to have a history of exposure to HPT; he found seventy-six. In any comparative study, whenever the number of abnormalities of any kind that are observed in a drug-exposed population is similar to the number that would be expected in an unexposed population, it is unlikely any of the abnormalities are drug-related. In Koller's large study the results were completely negative and totally out of line with those of Dr. Gal.

Koller discussed the obvious weakness in our study. GPs' records in the UK were not precise enough to enable us to place the estimated dates of exposure to drugs within the one-week time-bands that Koller had been able to do for German women. To be sure of demonstrating a relationship between a drug and the type of abnormality that it might have caused, it is essential to know the precise dates of exposure and relate them to the stage in the development of that organ. The development of almost all the vital organs is completed within the first six weeks. We had only been able to sort our cases crudely into three groups, dividing the nine months of pregnancy into three-month periods called trimesters – first "trimester" (conception to end of month three) – and so on. Many of the

HPT exposures in our cases, and in Dr Gal's series, had been too late to have caused spina bifida even if HPT had been a teratogen. Professor Koller was sure that the modest excess of exposures in our study would turn out merely to reflect the previous history of abnormalities among the women or their families. A pregnancy test was more likely to have been done in a woman with such a history so she could have an early termination if there was likely to be another abnormality. Koller warned that any new UK scheme would fail unless the quality of medical records was considerably improved. His advice dampened my enthusiasm for expanding or even continuing the CSD study.

Towards the end of 1978 an Association for Children Damaged by Hormone Pregnancy Tests was formed with the intention of securing compensation from Schering Chemicals Ltd, the manufacturers of Primodos. It would be extremely difficult to obtain compensation for individual children when there was no way of confirming that the damage was due to HPT rather than some other factor. It is unwise to raise the hopes of anxious parents of damaged children unless there is scientific proof that a drug is the cause of abnormalities. Understandably emotions run high whenever there is a possibility that avoidable damage has occurred, especially to a child.

A test case had been brought against Schering. I was not directly involved but was asked to review all the published work touching on HPT which might be produced in court. I assessed ninety-eight studies from the world literature. Twenty-one papers had suggested a possible link with abnormalities of various kinds, forty-one had shown no effect and the remaining thirty-six were merely anecdotes contributing little one way or the other. It was noteworthy that the twenty-one publications tending to support the case against HPT had come from only ten groups of authors and several of the papers covered the same patients. Apart from Dr. Gal (who published three of the twenty-one papers) none of the other publications had pointed specifically to spina bifida. In common with several other expert witnesses who had been asked to assess the same material, I considered that no risk of HPT had been confirmed.

I agreed that my report could be shared with lawyers working on another US case. They were representing Ortho Pharmaceuticals and a gynaecologist, Dr. Crawley, who were being sued by the mother of a child who had been born with spina bifida. This case was to take Dr. Gal and a number of UK experts to a court room in Chattanooga, Tennessee. It was to be a memorable experience I will relate in some detail because I learned much about the pitfalls and devious legal procedures that apply in US litigation.

I spent a tedious and very hot week in the Chattanooga Choo-Choo Hilton Hotel waiting to be called to the trial. I saw a little of Chattanooga during the weekend and met the lawyers occasionally for progress reports. The reason for the long incarceration in my hotel was that the timing of my appearance was apparently critical to the defence's presentation. I was called towards the end of the week and spent nearly five hours "on the stand" (where the witness sits). The atmosphere in court was relaxed and at one point I addressed the elderly judge, Frank W. Wilson as "Your Worship," hastily correcting it to "Your Honour," which pleased him immensely. The defence case was lead by Mr. Robert Hardin, an extremely knowledgeable and likeable Southerner who had an incredible depth of understanding of the case and the scientific controversies surrounding it.

Bob Hardin opened with a number of questions about my work and how the Committee on Safety of Medicines operated. He questioned me about the Gal article, what we had thought of it in 1967 and why I had encouraged her to publish it even though the Committee was quite unconvinced by her evidence. I said I was sure Dr. Gal was totally sincere in her belief that HPT caused spina bifida. She had accused the

Committee, the Department and myself of "stonewalling." I explained that the reasons for our apparent lack of response to her preliminary results were, firstly, we had not been convinced by them and secondly, and more important, that any precipitate action by the Committee could have been alarming for women who had used oral contraceptives or had been treated with hormones for a menstrual disorder. Her second more detailed paper had appeared in 1972, five years after the first, but turned out to be little more than a rehash of the original data. Mr. Hardin then asked a key question - "Should the Committee or Minister have taken action after Gal's second paper?" I replied:

> "In view of what I have just said about the spin-off into other forms of treatment, I think it would have been irresponsible to recommend dramatic action at that point. It is the coward's way out to take action and perhaps bask in the reflected glory of the newspapers for doing something positive against a drug. It takes more courage to exercise restraint, and I vigorously defend my colleagues and former colleagues on the Committee and in the Department of Health in taking no action at that stage."

We moved on to describe the Committee's study I had designed and in which my colleague Dr. Gill Greenberg (no relation to Martin Greenberg, chapter three) had played a leading part. Hardin referred to several earlier witnesses who had used the word "association" to describe relations between drugs and abnormalities. He wanted me to say whether, if there was an "association" between the use of a drug and a subsequent abnormality, this was the same as a "causal association." Did it mean that the drug had *caused* the abnormality? The court had spent a long time on this point and he asked me to try to explain this vitally important distinction to the jury in my own words. A glance at the jury suggested that the answer would have to be in words they would understand rather than words I would normally have used. I contrived a metaphor I hoped might illustrate this important difference. I told them that in England we paint most of our mail-boxes red. It would be easy to perform a study proving a statistically significant *association* between the colour red and mail-boxes, but this did not mean painting something red turns it into a mail-box. The lawyers told me later they believed most of the jurors had understood this for the first time in the trial. It was extremely important because in studies such as ours, and for that matter Dr. Gal's, it is possible to prove many statistically valid associations that are not causal associations. A woman might have taken several drugs during her pregnancy. All the drugs, all the family details, all the woman's medical history, her particular occupation, smoking and drinking habits were factors that could be associated with the abnormality but were probably not a cause of it.

Hardin asked me give examples of factors that might have influenced perception of the results of the studies. I said that several of the authors had published the same results in more than one journal and might have created the impression there was more support for the HPT hypothesis than was justified. I suggested that *positive results bias* might have been a particularly important source of misunderstanding in this case. Editors tend to accept papers describing a new hazard and reject those that confirm safety. I remembered one of the examples quoted by my friend David Sackett of McMaster University in Canada. David collected biases with the same enthusiasm some people collect stamps. I used his example of the bias introduced by topicality. He called it "hot stuff" bias. Editors are influenced by the topicality of the subject when they have to decide whether to give space to it. If, on the other hand, someone shows something is safe, they will use their limited space for a more interesting story. David called this positive results bias. (Many wished there was a "Journal of Negative Results" which would print such papers). Analyses based merely on the number of publications are often misleading. This was one reason why I was suspicious of the so-called "meta-analysis" that was a rather new "buzz" word in those days. My own assessment of nearly a hundred papers on HPT might have been described as a meta-analysis, but I did not claim it had been possible to compare the various works in a scientifically acceptable way. Few of the authors had used the same methods, most suffered from missing data and almost none of them had been able to compare like-with-like. I also suggested that memory or recall bias could be a devastating source of trouble. Mothers of abnormal babies would be far more likely to remember details and be able to answer questions about their pregnancy than the mothers of normal babies. Recall bias tends to make case records more detailed than control records. I was extremely dubious about any retrospective studies not based on written medical records that had been created before the investigation started. I was especially critical of the "telephone-interview" technique so often used in the US where the interviewer may be unable to avoid unconscious bias creeping into the interrogation. I could not forget the story about early social survey that had been conducted on the telephone at a time only rich people could afford a telephone!

Bob Hardin then set up a screen and I showed graphs of the UK rates for births of babies with limb deformities and sales of thalidomide. The rates of abnormalities had started to rise nine months after the drug was first marketed and fell after it was withdrawn. I showed the corresponding graphs for HPT sales and the deformity rates showing no change even though the sales of HPT had increased dramatically. Finally, Hardin asked me if, after examining the plaintiff's records, I could find any evidence that HPT could have caused the plaintiff's spina bifida. According to the dates in the medical records, she had been exposed to HPT at six weeks of gestation. This was too late to have caused the gross abnormalities in the unfortunate child's spine. After a ten minute recess the Court resumed and the proceedings started to get rather more robust. I shall quote from the transcript prepared by the court stenographer on a shorthand writing machine which encodes the exchanges verbatim on a continuous roll of paper.

Mr. Dick Jahn, for the plaintiff, started his cross-examination by asking me if I agreed that nearly all epidemiological studies had defects. Of course, I did. He then said,

> "If I came to you and said 'name your price, I have got to do a hatchet job on a series of epidemiological reports,' you could give me a lot of ammunition on how to attack them, couldn't you?"

I replied I had no experience of doing "hatchet jobs," but I could give many examples of how bias can affect studies, especially when the events being studied are rare. Mr. Jahn then, for reasons that are not clear in the court transcript, tried to switch the dialogue to the work I had done on thrombosis and oral contraceptives. This had nothing to do with the case that had brought me to Chattanooga. He succeeded in confusing me and I am sure the jury, but perhaps this was all part of the process of softening up the witness. He switched back to the question of association versus causation and tried to get me to agree that if thalidomide had been associated with abnormalities and had also been the cause, Isabel Gal's demonstration of an association must mean that HPT had also caused the abnormalities! Jahn asked me if I would give HPT or similar hormones to a pregnant woman, and when I said "No, because it is not necessary," he tried to persuade the jury that I was saying this because I feared they were teratogenic. I added that if an obstetrician saw some need to use a hormone mixture in a pregnant woman, I would have no worry about any risk it would produce spina bifida.

Having exhausted this line of attack, Jahn tried another ruse to "impeach" me, which I understand is frequently resorted to by cross-examining lawyers in an attempt to damage the credibility of witness.

Jahn: Now, Doctor, you started your career with some
         thing that is called ICI, or something of that sort?
Inman: Yes.
Jahn: Were you working with this company when a
         drug known as clofibrate was developed?
Inman: Yes.
Jahn: Later you were with the Committee on Safety of
         Drugs?
Inman: Yes. (What is he driving at? I wondered)
Jahn: You supported that drug against the evidence of a
         massive World Health Organisation trial?

Now as they say, I had him "over a barrel." He was referring to a large study by the WHO which had suggested some adverse effects of clofibrate. It had been heavily criticised by a number of prominent epidemiologists. I had no involvement whatsoever in the WHO study. On August 2nd, 1982 in a letter published by Colin Johnson and Arabella Melville titled "Drugs under the influence" which discussed the structure of the CSM and its civil servants, they had said:

"The number of people available for all the bodies and institutions requiring experts is limited. Dr. Bill Inman's career illustrates this merry-go-round. He worked for ICI when a cholesterol-lowering drug, clofibrate, was being developed there; later, as Principal

Medical Officer at the CSM, he supported the drug against the evidence of a massive WHO trial."

Inman: I know exactly what you are getting at Mr. Jahn; you are referring to a letter in *The Guardian* by Arabella Melville. She had discovered a chapter in my textbook that disagreed with the WHO findings on clofibrate. The chapter was written by J. I. Mann, not by Bill Inman! She wrongly attributed this statement to me.

I produced the book from my brief-case and held it up for the Jury to see while Mr Jahn started to go red in the face.

Jahn: Well, I guess I really stepped into that one! Can I sue *The Guardian,* Doctor? (laughter)

Back to the main topic of the Committee's warning, I was asked if I would reiterate the Committee's views. I said;

"Firstly, we did not believe that HPT was teratogenic. Secondly, we did not want to draw undue attention to Dr. Gal's paper and give it too much weight because of the bad effects this might have on women who were using the pill. Thirdly, we were aware that the indication had been removed from Schering's literature. Some people argued about this decision, but a lot of people were involved in it and that was their decision."

Mr. Jahn said that the Committee had put out a warning within days of the publicity generated by Dr. Gal and Oliver Gillie. I disagreed, pointing out it would have taken the Committee six to eight weeks to have the warning statement drafted, agreed by them, checked, printed and distributed. We had started this process several weeks before The *Sunday Times* article. Mr. Jahn then went on to imply that ever since that time I had borne a grudge against Isabel Gal. I replied:

> "I have never felt unkindly towards Dr. Gal. We have, as it happens, just met in the corridor and shaken hands and greeted each other as old friends and colleagues. I think she is wrong, she thinks I am wrong, but that has nothing to do with whether I like her or not."

I left the courtroom almost disappointed that the Plaintif's case seemed to have so little scientific content.

The end of the trial was dramatic. The day after I had given evidence I flew back to England without waiting for the verdict. Before it was delivered Judge Wilson suffered a fatal heart attack! A mis-trial was declared. I believe the verdict would have gone to the defendants, but the trial had proved to be so expensive that the case was abandoned.

7   A Plethora of Committees

The mid-Seventies brought me into uncomfortable contact with a problem that spawned a shoal of subcommittees and working parties – the safety of whooping-cough vaccine. In 1967 the Department of Health had decided the CSM's yellow card scheme should be used to report adverse reactions to vaccines as well as drugs. This involved liaison with its Joint Committee on Vaccination and Immunisation (JCVI). It was a departure from our normal rules of confidentiality in the sense we had previously promised doctors that under no circumstances would the yellow cards be shown to anybody outside the Committee's Secretariat unless their names and those of their patients had been obscured. Photocopies of the cards were now to be passed to the JCVI. Up to that time I had assured audiences on public platforms I would not show a yellow card in its original form even to Sir George Godber, the Chief Medical Officer. The cards were addressed to the Committee, not the Department of Health. Faced with this instruction from above I had tried to justify the change by explaining that the secretariat of the JCVI could be regarded as an extension of our own. I hoped the JCVI would appreciate the damage that could be done to the yellow card system if confidentiality of identities was breached by them. Nevertheless I was horrified at one meeting, shortly after I had returned from a holiday, to see an open document case belonging to one of the participants at a meeting of one of the vaccine committees. It was overflowing with photocopies of yellow cards with the names of doctors and patients clearly visible. The case belonged to an employee of one of the drug manufacturers. I had certainly not authorised such a release of confidential information; presumably officials from some other department had helped themselves to the documents while I was on leave.

Whether the whooping cough vaccine had reduced the incidence of whooping cough had been hotly argued for many years. There had also been considerable concern about its safety because some children had suffered severe brain damage after vaccination. Critics of the vaccine programme referred to the profound reduction in the disease recorded before the vaccine had been introduced. Between 1950 and 1975 there had been eight epidemics of whooping cough at roughly three-year intervals, each one smaller than the one preceding it. In 1951 there had been about sixty-five thousand notifications. In successive epidemics the numbers had dropped to fifty thousand, thirty thousand and twenty thousand respectively and then in the next four epidemics to ten thousand or less.[35] The national immunisation programme, however, had been started only after the third of these epidemics had already passed its peak and could therefore have played no large part in the already massive reduction which had been recorded. There had also been a tenfold reduction in deaths from whooping-cough from a total of about one thousand each year to about one hundred, again before the vaccination programme had been started. This dramatic reduction in whooping cough morbidity and mortality mainly reflected better post-war housing and nutrition. In spite of this, the JCVI were convinced the low incidence could be attributed, at least in part, to the vaccine. They recommended the vaccination programme should continue but very prudently warned that infants with a history of epilepsy or any other central nervous illness should not be immunised against whooping-cough.

Much of the credit for putting pressure on the Department to reconsider the safety of the vaccine must go to a member of the public, Mrs. Rosemary Fox, whose daughter had been severely brain-damaged after immunisation, and to Jack Ashley, the founder and champion of the Association of Parents of Vaccine Damaged Children (APVDC). The JCVI had responded by setting up a Subcommittee on the Complications of Vaccination (SCV) to examine the reports of adverse reactions. Perhaps because the members of this subcommittee regarded themselves as the experts, or perhaps because some of them really were THE experts, they largely ignored the reports of reactions collected by the Committee on Safety of Medicines. They seemed not to be interested in the CSM's contribution even though we had been collecting and assessing the data for more than seven years.

Two years before the SCV had been established I had reviewed all the CSM's reports. This had turned out to have been a very useful exercise, prompted by the need to answer more than seventy parliamentary questions from Jack Ashley about the safety of whooping-cough vaccine. At least we were well aware of the problem, even if we had no means of telling him how large it was. We had twenty reports of encephalitis (brain inflammation) and sixty-eight of convulsions; fifteen children had died. This was a small incidence when considering the numbers of children vaccinated over the seven year period from 1967 when we first asked doctors to use the yellow cards for vaccines. Convulsions are not uncommon during infancy and some would have happened anyway. Another factor made assessment very difficult; the whooping-cough vaccine was often combined with vaccines for diphtheria and tetanus, the so-called Triple Vaccine, and sometimes with polio as well, the Quadruple Vaccine. Frequently it was not possible to decide which of the three or four components might have been responsible for a reaction, assuming any of them had. I advised the Department that our experience with other drugs suggested it was because very few of the serious reactions that had occurred had been reported. Those reported might be less than ten per cent of those that had occurred. This became painfully true when I had the opportunity to examine the very much larger number of APVDC reports from Mrs. Fox, almost none of which had been reported independently to our Committee.

Mrs. Fox's APVDC sent us details of more than five hundred and fifty children known to have developed severe reactions. Two hundred and forty of these cases were well documented and, by themselves, amounted to three times the number already reported to the Committee from all other sources. The remainder of the notifications comprised only the names and addresses of children with alleged reactions to the vaccine but gave no details. In April 1977 I wrote a paper proposing a strategy for investigating them and included a preliminary opinion on the first sixty records supplied by Mrs. Fox. I concluded that most of the children had definitely been damaged by the vaccine. Mrs. Fox's reports were much more detailed than the brief summaries we had collected from GPs. While many of the reports to the CSM described cases with very mild symptoms, all the APVDC children had been hospitalised and most had been assessed by brain specialists. The majority had residual disability ranging from weakness or convulsions to idiocy or a persistent vegetative state. Most of the parents had been told at the hospitals that the vaccine was the probable cause of the damage. Where the parents' correspondence was included, the general tone was one of dignified acceptance of their child's misfortune, concern about their care in later life and anxiety about the safety of other children. Surprisingly few parents hinted at litigation and the few criticisms of doctors or other medical staff related to obvious mismanagement. In many cases communication between nurses giving the injections, parents and general practitioners had failed. Children who had developed a temperature or had screamed repeatedly or had muscular spasms or convulsions after the first injection, had sometimes been given further doses of vaccine with catastrophic results.

My plan for the investigation was simply to send our field officers around to interview the medical staff involved with each child, starting with the recent reports where the details were likely to be most fresh, and working backwards in time. One weekend I drafted briefing letters for immediate use by our field officers, but I did not distribute them because the officials insisted the letters and forms should be approved by all the committees involved with the vaccine problem. This delayed the start of the follow up. I was then called into the Under Secretary's office and carpeted for the delay in starting the investigation that had left his officials vulnerable to criticism by the Minister! By the end of 1977 eight separate groups were involved, each insisting that copies of the documentation should be sent to them. On one occasion I stormed up to the "top of the office" to complain about a rumour I had overheard that my long-suffering secretary, Alice Renauld, had slipped up on the job of preparing all the copies. The list of committees, sub-committees and working parties looking at this one problem almost beggars belief; it comprised:

1. the Joint Committee on Vaccination and Immunisation,
2. its Sub-Committee on Vaccine Reactions,
3. the Committee on Safety of Medicines ,
4. its Subcommittee on Adverse Reactions,
5. a working party appointed by the CSM chaired by Dr. Tom Meade of the MRC,
6. a special Vaccine Advisory Panel chaired by the late Professor Dudgeon,
7. a group advising the APVDC,
8. a group headed by Professor Miller at the Middlesex Hospital who were embarking on a National Childhood Encephalopathy Study.

The small number of reports to the CSM amounted to only one serious reaction per three-hundred-thousand children vaccinated. This represented the reported incidence, and it was almost certainly only a small fraction, probably less than one tenth, of the real incidence. This low figure was seized on by the administrators as a politically convenient one which could be used to defend the Department's forthcoming publicity campaign to promote the use of the vaccine. In other situations when eager to ban a drug or put pressure on a drug company, the officials would have argued quite differently. They would have emphasised it was probable that only one in ten reactions had been reported and it was therefore necessary to multiply the number of reports by ten to estimate the risk. By this time I had examined the first eighty of Mrs. Fox's cases and found only one had also been reported to the Committee by the patient's doctor! If this was typical of all the reports, it suggested only one or two per cent of the cases might have been reported. It was also quite possible Mrs. Fox's group had only assembled a small fraction of the reactions that had occurred. My "informed guess" was that the likely incidence of serious reactions was about one in thirty thousand and certainly not one in three hundred thousand.

By the end of September 1977 I had been able to assess all but sixteen of the two hundred and forty documented APVDC cases. I concluded that one hundred and sixty-seven (three-quarters of them) had probably been caused by or aggravated by the vaccine. When added to the cases reported independently to the CSM, the incidence of serious complications seemed likely to be at least one in thirty thousand (and even this could be an under-estimate). It was at least ten times higher than the figure of one in three hundred thousand that the Department was clinging to.

On October 19th 1977 the Chief Medical Officer, Sir Henry Yellowlees, wrote to all doctors to advise them about the campaign soon to be launched to promote vaccination. Two days later I made one more attempt to avert what seemed to be a potential disaster and Dr. Diana Walford, a colleague who had also looked at the APVDC cases together with even more material provided by Professor Gordon Stewart from Glasgow, also wrote in strong support of my memorandum. Diana was destined to become a Deputy Chief Medical Officer at the Department. Professor Gordon Stewart, who was one of the best opinions on vaccine safety in the UK, had been invited by the APVDC to conduct an independent assessment of their case-material and it was proposed he should join Professor Dudgeon's Advisory Panel. This had been vetoed by Dudgeon. His antipathy to Gordon Stewart had led to the formation of yet another group to consider the whooping-cough vaccine problem. The conflict boiled over during one of the meetings. I had never before seen anybody so shoddily treated as Gordon was and the incident left a bad taste in my mouth for many months.

At this point I was immobilised by a prolonged strike of engineers who refused to repair the office lift on which I depended at work. I could not expect colleagues to carry my heavy wheelchair and me up several flight of stairs, so I had to work at home. However, our concern about the incidence of vaccine reactions at last had some effect and Sir Henry sent a second letter to all doctors on November 24th advising them the media campaign had been cancelled. The vaccine would still be available but he stressed the great importance of avoiding its use in conditions that might make children unduly sensitive. I was not popular with the lay officials and was rather glad to be out of London.

By the end of 1977 I finished the assessment of the case-reports. Nobody seemed to disagree with the clinical assessment, only with my uncomfortable conclusion that the incidence of serious reactions was at least ten times larger than the officially admitted figure. The CSM's Advisory Panel would not be able to complete its work until the end of

1979. I had done all I could reasonably do with the material available to me and was more than happy to concentrate on other matters, especially my plans for an independent monitoring unit.

In their final report, the Advisory Panel, who now had more accurate estimates of the quantity of vaccine injected, based their estimates of the risk of whooping-cough vaccination on three and a half million children who had received a total of ten and a half million injections. After studying the cases (the same material I had already studied) they arrived at a figure for serious central nervous system side-effects of one in twenty-nine thousand! Their estimate for the risk of permanent brain damage was one in fifty-four thousand. They regarded these as minimum risks because of the likelihood of under-reporting. I was too angry to feel smug that their conclusions coincided precisely with mine.

The vaccination of very young children, who may be at almost no risk themselves, to produce "herd" immunity, raises moral and ethical issues that do not seem to have been properly addressed. If the Department of Health promotes what almost looks like compulsory medication by putting pressure on doctors and mothers to participate in national programmes, it must ensure that any damaged child is adequately cared for. Nowadays this will require a seven figure sum if it is to guarantee life-long support for each severely disabled child and not the derisory sums being paid so far. Large sums should not, in my view, be paid directly to parents as "compensation" but set aside for local authorities to provide care throughout the victim's life and not only while parents are alive. There has been talk of removing patients from doctors' lists if they do not comply with instructions about the vaccination of their children. If this became the rule, there would be no residual doubt about the element of compulsion. Nobody can doubt the wisdom of smallpox vaccination, the only programme that has ever eliminated a disease world-wide. No-one can doubt the wisdom of vaccinating against polio, when the incidence of permanent damage after an attack is so large. However, should a healthy child, living in conditions in which it is almost certain to survive an attack by one or more of the childhood epidemics without residual damage, be vaccinated? Should it be placed at risk for the benefit of other children who may be at greater risk? Should a schoolgirl be vaccinated against rubella to protect the offspring of others when there may be no guarantee their immunity will last until she starts to rear her own family? A woman who is contemplating pregnancy could be tested to see if she has escaped immunity from natural disease and then be vaccinated before she gets pregnant.

Shortly before leaving the Department in 1980, I was told by a senior official I had "seriously damaged my career" during these studies by criticising the Department's position on the safety of the whooping cough vaccine and possibly causing embarrassment to the Minister. When I reacted angrily by suggesting that whoever had said it should do something unmentionable to a rolling doughnut, this was hastily retracted, but a good friend in the Department told me "You know Bill, you've blown your K (for the "mini-pill" and developing the yellow card scheme) by daring to question the party line." It would not be the last time my distaste for expediency and compromise would get me into trouble with a system which uses the honours system to manipulate its advisers. I had never had a "K" on my personal agenda, though the title for June that would go with it might have been a small public recognition of the many sacrifices she had to make through the intrusion by my work on family life throughout these turbulent years.

8 Birth of the DSRU

In October 1970, three hundred delegates assembled at the National Academy of Sciences in Washington for a conference on Adverse Reactions Reporting Systems.[36] The speakers from the United Kingdom included Sir Derrick Dunlop, Jim Crooks, Martin Vessey and myself. The conference was billed as "International" but apart from ourselves and two speakers from the World Health Organisation in Geneva, almost all the participants were from the United States Food and Drug Administration (FDA) or the US pharmaceutical industry. Our task was to define the requirements for a National Centre for Drug Surveillance in the United States. At the top of the agenda was the vexed question of whether such a centre should be governmental or independent. On this fundamental issue the conference reported that:

> "Location within the FDA might pose a problem of maintaining scientific integrity of a Centre that is attempting to acquire new information on drugs while tied to a regulatory function. Fears could arise that reports will be biased to suit the needs of the regulators. This could apply, in general, to any location except that of a free-standing and isolated agency."

Accepting, however, that there was then no practical alternative to location within the FDA, the Conference went on to recommend:

"Neither the Director nor the staff of the Centre should participate in regulatory decisions. Their charge will be to seek and
collect both emerging and conclusive information about the
risk of drug use. They must be free to seek the truth wherever
that may lie. Regulations, however, must often stem from arbi-
trary decisions based on information available at a given time.
Thus direct involvement in regulatory decisions may be contradictory to the scientific role of the Centre's staff, and such
involvement must be absolutely avoided."

This recommendation contained a very clear message that many government agencies continue to ignore. It encapsulated the difficulty of recruiting quality staff and shielding them from political interference which had
been experienced by the FDA and other countries, and was anticipated in
my private discussions with Derrick Dunlop six years earlier. The
Conference proposed that the Centre would develop programmes for
intensive surveillance, including an improved spontaneous voluntary
reporting system, and would pay special attention to research into reactions which might take a very long time to appear. The asthma experience in the UK had illustrated the importance of continuous surveillance
of disease statistics and of linking them with changes in drug use. There
was also a great need for improved mechanisms for dissemination of
information to doctors and patients.

The conference identified the main defects in existing systems and it
is important to remember it preceded the Eraldin incident by nearly four
years. Thalidomide and Eraldin were never a problem in the US because
new drugs take longer to penetrate their regulatory screen and they were
not marketed there. Speedy passage of new drug applications (NDAs)
has been trumpeted as the "Jewel in the Crown" of the UK system.
However, several drug accidents in the UK could have been avoided by

the imposition of more rigid criteria and more intensive scrutiny before granting a licence.

When the Medicines Control Agency (MCA) was established to manage regulatory activities in the United Kingdom, it was set the seemingly incompatible tasks of both promoting the UK pharmaceutical industry and assuring drug safety. As predicted at the Washington meeting, great difficulty was experienced in recruiting a suitable director for the agency who was prepared to take this on. Eventually, in 1989, one was found – Dr. Keith Jones – experienced as a toxicologist in both agricultural chemicals and pharmaceuticals in various companies and who was currently working for a drug company in the United States. MCA actions that will be described later show what happens when medical issues associated with drug safety become confused with official attitudes to the commercial aspects of drug marketing. Every word of the recommendations of the Washington meeting was prophetic.

It has been said I was the first to use the acronym "PMS" (Post-Marketing Surveillance) to describe the various methods needed for monitoring the safety of new drugs. Whether this is true is immaterial but I remember talking about the need for PMS at an international conference at Wembley in 1965 and, as I left the lecture hall and wheeled myself through a trade exhibition, I passed a poster advertising in two-foot letters – "THE ANSWER TO PMS!" This probably stood for Post-Menopausal or pre-menstrual Syndrome and I remember joking to a colleague about "instant plagiarism." Some people are fond of inventing new names for old ideas. Civil servants and people seeking research grants are particularly prone to it. Currently the smart word is "pharmacovigilance," copied from the French presumably to conform with the European Community. It presumably means nothing more than being alert about drugs. I shall use the more descriptive Post-Marketing Surveillance (PMS). I am not very fond of acronyms because they often have several meanings and I tend to get them mixed up. Recently we have been introduced to "EBM" (Evidence-based Medicine). When I was doing my obstetrics forty-five years ago it stood for Expressed Breast Milk, was kept in the ward fridge and occasionally served in the coffee to unsuspecting housemen!

Although the Washington conference had pointed the way, no progress in PMS was made in the UK for several years. In the US, Herschel Jick, Sidney Shapiro and the late Dennis Sloan set up the Boston Collaborative Drug Surveillance Program (BCDSP). It was very successful, but local and limited to a number of hospitals in Massachusetts in which data were collected by "Nurse Monitors." In the UK in 1974, Eraldin reminded us vividly that safety must not depend on the vagaries of spontaneous reporting to a government agency. The yellow card system was in place but few used it because the events were difficult to distinguish as adverse reaction. Even if they were identified there were various other deterrents to reporting. What was needed was a new scheme that would record events irrespective of doctors' suspicions that they might have been caused by a drug.

I was the first person to set up such a system on a national scale in the UK, but I was not the first to point to the important differences between an event that might have occurred anyway and one that was an adverse reaction to a drug. This was defined by Professor David Finney of the Department of Statistics at the University of Aberdeen three months before I joined the Committee to develop the voluntary reporting (yellow card) system in 1964.[37] Although not a medical man (which might be regarded as a positive advantage), David retained an unflagging interest in all aspects of drug-safety monitoring and was still, thirty years later, an active member of the Trust now managing the Drug Safety Research Unit (DSRU) that I had founded in Southampton in 1980. David defined an event as

"A particular untoward happening experienced by a patient, undesirable either generally or in the context of his disease.

The term is not to be limited either to recognised side-effects of a drug or to incidents that are in some sense unexpected. Every patient in the monitor field to whom an event occurs will be noted, irrespective of whether that event is thought to be wholly or partly caused by the drug."

His paper remains the clearest description of the principles upon which a national monitoring system should be based and is required reading for anybody interested in drug safety work. Unfortunately his far-reaching proposals were largely ignored by the Department until the Eraldin tragedy drew attention to the defects in the facilities it had provided. Another six years passed before I was able to put David's event-monitoring ideas into effect, and to do this I had to set up an independent institution outside the Department of Health.

Throughout 1975 I worked on an idea for a new monitoring method that I called "Recorded Release." The first opportunity to debate it arose at a large and rather unusual conference in Hawaii in January 1976. The thirty-seven speakers included many of the most experienced people in drug monitoring from ten countries. The cross-cultural East-West Centre in Honolulu had been set up by the Japanese and American governments to provide low-cost conference facilities within easy reach of both countries. The conference was called to discuss existing and future drug monitoring methods with Japanese experts who were investigating a massive "epidemic" of a disease of the nervous system suspected to be due to a drug called clioquinol that was sold worldwide for the treatment of "traveller's diarrhoea." The problem seemed to be largely confined to Japan. The disease was called subacute myelo-optico-neuropathy. It was hardly surprising that everyone referred to it by its acronym "SMON."

I chaired the first session on drug-monitoring systems and was also the first speaker. My main themes were the low efficiency of spontaneous reporting schemes and the need for more sophisticated methods. I listed the "Seven Deadly Sins" that had been suggested to explain why the adverse reaction reporting rate was so inadequate. The first, complacency, was the mistaken belief that only safe drugs are licensed for use. The second, fear of litigation, was not much of a disincentive to reporting in the UK because few doctors are sued by their patients, but is a major concern in the US where litigation is almost a national sport and is the first thought of anyone who suffers an injury. The third was a sense of guilt for having caused harm. The fourth was ambition to collect and publish a personal series of cases; this can delay general awareness of a serious hazard and is probably one of the worst of the sins. The fifth sin was ignorance of the mechanism for reporting suspected reactions, largely due to inadequate publicity by the CSM. The sixth was diffidence about reporting a mere suspicion; doctors might fear ridicule. Finally the last of the deadly sins was lethargy or indifference to the doctor's responsibility to contribute to the general advancement of knowledge.[38] Over-riding all these was the great difficulty in distinguishing drug reactions from events that would have happened anyway, including complications of the disease for which the patient was being treated.

It was suggested that all new drugs should undergo a period of monitoring by the manufacturers. All records of suspected reactions would be sent to the authorities. Several schemes had been tried but, however well-meaning, the efforts of company medical staff were often frustrated by their sales colleagues to whom the procedure was seen as a barrier to rapid expansion of sales. As we shall see later, however, many sales departments began to see PMS in an entirely different light. They woke up to the fact that it could be used as an opportunity for active promotion. Once a GP had agreed to take part in a PMS study, the "rep" would have a guaranteed entrée to the surgery for as long as he could prolong the illusion that the doctor was contributing to scientific knowledge. My

Recorded Release scheme would be conducted by the Committee on Safety of Medicines rather than the drug companies. Immediately after a new drug had been licensed and until the Committee was satisfied that it had an acceptable level of safety, doctors would only be permitted to prescribe the new drug if they agreed to complete a follow-up form committing them to a period of close observation. The drugs selected for this scheme would be called "Recorded drugs." When prescribing one of them, the doctor would be required to record the patient's name and address and the date of first treatment and to send these details to the Committee at the time of prescribing. Subsequently he would have to send further cards at three-monthly intervals, usually for a year. If a potential hazard was "signalled," the period of monitoring could be extended. Although it could not have prevented it completely, the scheme should have identified the problem with Eraldin long before such large numbers of patients had suffered serious adverse reactions. Obviously companies would resist the idea because it would slow the growth in the early sales of the new product.

I anticipated that whatever form of "PMS" was adopted, it might be difficult to brief GPs so they understood the difference between an adverse reaction and an adverse event as defined by David Finney. When I modified the original proposals for Recorded Release to a less complicated scheme that I called Prescription-Event Monitoring (PEM), more than 1,500,000 questionnaires were distributed to doctors, each bearing the following message:

"A broken leg is an EVENT. If more fractures were associated with this drug they could have been due to hypotension, central nervous system effects or metabolic bone changes."

There can be no denying that a broken leg is an "event"; a very painful one. A drug might have lowered a patient's blood pressure excessively or caused loss of co-ordination and made her unsteady on her feet or it might have caused excessive loss of calcium from the bones and softened them. This simple expression of David Finney's idea successfully eliminated most of the confusion that would otherwise have arisen when the scheme was started five years later.

In April 1976 I repeated my Honolulu presentation at the 83rd Congress of the Royal Society of Health in Eastbourne.[39] My Recorded Release package was now rather more sophisticated and comprised a prescription-kit resembling a cheque-book personalised for each patient. The prototype kits included a pink form for notifying the Committee that the first prescription had been issued and four green forms to be stored in the patient's notes and posted at three-month intervals. The scheme was simple and could be easily adapted to suit the computer systems being introduced into general practice. The problem would be to persuade the Department to provide the resources required to operate it and the doctors to use it.

In January 1977, exactly a year after the first Honolulu conference, I returned to the East-West Centre to present the latest version of the scheme in more detail. The conference, like the first, was sponsored by Ciba-Geigy and most ably organised by one of their doctors, Oliver Pinto, who had played a very significant role behind the scenes for several years, encouraging people in many countries to take more interest in PMS. Oliver appreciated better than most that the key to safety lay in the development of monitoring schemes free from political and commercial influence. He believed, as I did, that the companies should not attempt to conduct PMS studies themselves. He recognised that an independent agency would need "no-strings" financial support from the industry since it was very unlikely any health department would support a costly national system over which it had no control. The majority of new drugs would prove to have an acceptable margin of safety which would be good news for the companies. Early detection of hazards would protect patients from continued risk and at the same time protect the industry from discredit and litigation. Oliver believed I could persuade companies that they could be in a "no lose" position if they supported an independent non-governmental institution.

Forty-five delegates from eleven government agencies, eighteen universities and five drug companies attended the second Honolulu conference. This was the most experienced and innovative group in drug safety monitoring ever assembled under one roof before or since. It is sad to reflect today that, with very few exceptions, there has been virtually no real progress in the majority of countries, usually because they have been stifled by bureaucracy and poor funding or because young people of adequate calibre have not come forward to implement and expand the ideas, formulated twenty years ago, and to fill the gaps left by those who have left the scene.

The moving spirit behind this second conference was the late Franz Gross, Professor of Pharmacology in Heidelberg. Franz was a great friend and probably the best conference chairman I have ever met. Besides a far reaching knowledge of his subject, I have heard him converse fluently in six European languages and he had an unmatched ability to stimulate ideas, smooth ruffled feathers and sum up clearly. Franz was a "workaholic" who contributed significantly to the progress of drug safety monitoring for many years. One evening he was found, by his wife, dead at his desk. My paper on Recorded Release had been widely circulated before the conference and was published in the book of the conference that Franz and I jointly edited, but it was not put on sale until several people had jumped on the bandwagon and published papers proposing minor modifications of the Recorded Release scheme under slightly different titles.[40]

Although the Adverse Reactions Committee liked the idea that PMS should be developed along these lines, it had become very clear by 1978 that the management of the Licensing Authority was not going to support it and would prefer that the industry took over. Recorded Release as a function of the CSM was doomed. It would fail because of the adversarial situation so ably described by one of the participants at the Honolulu conference, Kenneth Hammond.[41] Ken was Professor of Social Psychology at the University of Boulder, Colorado, a pioneer of decision theory and an expert in research into the factors that shape industrial and political policy making. His presentation mirrored most of the problems I had encountered while trying to develop the yellow card system over sixteen difficult years.

Ken's starting point resembled the situation in 1964 when I first joined the Department. The role of scientists was supposed to be quite different from the role of policy makers. Scientists assemble the evidence and present it to the policy makers who decide the social policy and legislation to best serve the public. However, to use Ken's own words — "not only are these functions confused, but legislators and scientists exchange roles." Legislators demand that their scientific advisers should participate in policy-making and the scientists begin to enjoy involvement with prominent politicians and the media, and may even offer policy suggestions before being asked for them. He wrote:

"Scientists, therefore, do not passively provide facts and let the policy decisions fall where they may. When government officials invite them to influence legislation, scientists do not refuse, because they cannot refuse; the situation demands that they respond to the invitation. Unfortunately, in this way scientists who intend to serve merely as expert witnesses become policy advocates, and legislators frequently pit them against one another as opponents. In the process, scientists become incompetent amateur legislators at best, and self-serving advocates at worst."

The policy makers, in their turn, become interested in scientific matters and rapidly come to believe they know as much as or more than the scientists who are starting to argue with them. One of the consequences he said was "the greatest perversion of science – deliberate bias."

"On the other hand, the adversarial process makes amateur scientists out of legislators, because it requires them to focus on, and become interested in, the scientific aspects of problems. Instead of concerning themselves with the social values that should control the application of science and technology to social problems, they seek out details that enable them to do battle with scientists. Thus scientists become incompetent social legislators, and social legislators become incompetent scientists. No one benefits from this confusion."

I always tried to avoid being drawn into adversarial situations (sometimes described as "science courts") but the Hammond model accurately describes the relations between the medical and lay staff serving our various committees. When scientists become locked into the establishment, the tradition of "on tap but not on top" I described earlier in the context of oral contraception and whooping-cough vaccination, begins to take over. The issue, perhaps the draft answer to a Parliamentary Question, is usually decided by a hierarchy of non-scientists who believe they are the best judges of the situation. An Assistant Principal reports to a Principal and the messages travels up the ladder to a Senior Principal, an Assistant Secretary and an Under Secretary and eventually to the Minister who says what he is advised to say, often without being warned about the uncertainties and caveats that a scientific adviser would normally insist on.

The Minister was not the only person to be fed with sanitised information. Each committee meeting was preceded by a briefing meeting between the Chairman and senior officials. Each of these "pre-meeting meetings" was preceded by what I used to call the "What shall we tell the Chairman" meeting of civil servants. In fairness to the civil servants, with some Chairmen it was sometimes more a case of "What dare we tell the Chairman?" All the meetings and briefings took up a large portion of the time available to do the real job we were paid for − to assemble and assess the information.

Many years ago my deputy, the late Cliff Ruttle, remarked that "the Civil Service only recruits good innovators by accident." I did not fully appreciate what he meant at the time, but gradually came to realise that the service attracts people to their administrative grades who are not risk-takers and who tend therefore to be poor innovators. Most are content to keep their heads below the parapet and stick to the rules and traditions of the service. The turnover of medical staff in countries in which the drug safety monitoring centres have been located within government departments, has been rapid. It was once said that the "half-life" (the average time taken for half the staff to change jobs) of a doctor in the Food and Drug Administration in the US was eighteen months. In the UK I think it may have been a little longer, but my sixteen years in one job was exceptional. I had been lucky enough to be able to start something new and totally absorbing. I had no ambition for promotion to higher positions within the Department. I had been hired to set up a monitoring system for the Dunlop Committee and had done just that.

The relation between the Medicines Control Agency (MCA) and the pharmaceutical industry I touched on earlier in this chapter, has been discussed by Dr. Joe Collier, editor of the *Drug and Therapeutics Bulletin*[42], by Charles Medawar of Social Audit[43] and very recently by John Abraham of the University of Reading.[44] All three have pointed to the close and questionable relationship between the industry and the MCA. There has been an attempt to fuse two widely divergent functions – public safety assurance on the one hand and responsibility for protecting or promoting the interests of the pharmaceutical industry on the other. There can be few doubts about the need for the MCA to perform the first function but it would be more appropriate for the Department of Trade and Industry to supervise the commercial aspects of drug development. The scientific assessment of drug safety data should not be influenced in any way by the orders of the MCA's political masters. I shall comment later on the failure of the Department and its advisers to stop drug companies exploiting the gullibility and greed of doctors who take part in pseudo-scientific PMS studies which promote new drugs. When the Medicines Act of 1968 became effective in 1971, the regulatory authorities continued to focus on animal testing and clinical trials rather than finding the resources needed to study what happens when drugs are used on a large scale in everyday medical practice.

A large fraction of the NHS drug bill in general practice is spent on "me-too" drugs. "me-too" means "I want a share of the market." Drug company laboratories dissipate vast resources in the production of chemical variants of previously marketed drugs. Some of the β-blocking drugs promoted in the UK for angina and blood pressure are shown in Table I, and other examples among treatments for stomach ulcers, heart failure and angina and hypertension are shown in Table II. The lists do not include unbranded or "generic" preparations. Several companies formed other companies with names that give no clue as to their parentage. As the time approaches for the patent protection of a leading product to expire, the new company launches a "me too", apparently in competition with the parent company. So many closely related drugs are available that doctors cannot be expected to decide which is best or safest for their patient. GPs are almost totally dependent on the marketing ploys of the industry to determine what you and I get for our aching back or our angina. The literature that falls through doctors' doors or the interviews with salesmen often induce doctors to change treatment from drugs that have at least stood the test of time, to new "me too" drugs that may be equally effective (they are rarely more effective) but are an unknown quantity regarding safety until they have undergone a period of intensive independent post-marketing surveillance. The drugs listed in these tables reflect thousands of millions of dollars spent on largely unnecessary research, on patent filling and on submissions to government authorities in many countries. What is more important they also reflect the use of millions of "experimental" animals, thousands of human patients subjected to risk in largely unnecessary clinical trials, and tens of thousands who should be monitored carefully after licensing to assure that a "me-too" has a reasonable level of safety.

Although the risk may be small, every new drug is a potential "thalidomide" or "Eraldin." Small alterations in chemistry can have far-reaching effects. The manufacturers plead that unless they are allowed to replace their patent-expired products with new products and charge highly for them, they will not be able to raise the funds required to maintain their research into new classes of medicines or maintain their position as major contributors to the nation's wealth. In reality, most drug companies operating in the UK are foreign owned, and a very high proportion of their so-called research is nothing more than work on "me too" drugs! Why not change the patent laws so genuine new discoveries with proven clinical merit are protected indefinitely until displaced by genuinely innovative drugs which are significantly more effective? Extension of the patent life would make it less profitable to market "me too" products. It would also make it more difficult to justify high prices for many drugs in common use. With fewer products to distract doctors' attention, patients would almost certainly benefit. I would not be surprised if the national expenditure of some £4,500 million per annum could not be dramatically reduced, perhaps by as much as a half. It would, of course, be strongly opposed both by the industry and the MCA.

My forty years in medicine has spanned the introduction of approximately ninety-eight percent of all the drugs currently on the market. With very few exceptions, patients' needs for each type of drug – an NSAID for arthritis, a ß-blocker for heart disease, a tranquilliser and so on – can usually be met by the first two or three members of each chemical group of products produced. Antibiotics are noteworthy exceptions because bacteria develop resistance to them. The sixth, sixteenth or sixtieth copy-cat product is unlikely to have anything to offer apart from unknown dangers and they cost many times as much as the "generic copies" of the original products. Generic copies may be made by any company once the original patent has expired. A solution to this problem is easy to find. Doctors should prescribe one of the older members of each group of drugs until strong scientific evidence has been published in major medical journals supporting the claims for a new one. They should ignore most of the stories the company "reps" tell them and on no account should they agree to take part in any company-sponsored "PMS study." I shall explain why in chapter 10.

In 1978 I finally decided that if I wanted to improve the quality and efficiency of the "Safety Net" I would have to leave the Department and set up an independent unit. Although I could expect no help from the Licensing Authority, I received invaluable support from the late Dr Ed Harris, a Deputy Chief Medical Officer, and from the Department's Chief Scientist, Sir Douglas Black. There was a great deal to do during the next two years. I had to find a University that would be prepared to accommodate a self-financing institution and I had to raise funds. The medico-legal, ethical and confidentiality issues had to be debated at length with the British Medical Association, the General Medical Council, the Medical Research

Table I. The proliferation of Beta-blocking drugs in the treatment of hypertension

Approved Name	Brand Name	Drug Comany	Approved Name	Brand Name	Drug Comany
Acebutalol	Secadrex (2)	Rhone-Poulenc Rorer	Oxprenolol	Slow-Trasicor (1)	Ciba
"	Sectral (1)	Rhone-Poulenc Rorer	"	Trasicor (1)	Ciba
Atenolol	Beta-Adalat (2)	Bayer	"	Trasidrex (2)	Ciba
"	Kalten (3)	Zeneca	Pindolol	Viskaldix (2)	Sandoz
"	Tenben (2)	Galen	"	Visken (1)	Sandoz
"	Tenif (2)	Zeneca	Propraanolol	Beta-Prograne (1)	Tillomed
"	Tenoret 50 (2)	Zeneca	"	Inderal (1)	Zeneca (original ICI)
"	Tenoretic (2)	Zeneca	"	Inderetic (2)	Zeneca
"	Tenormin (1)	Zeneca	"	Inderex (2)	Zeneca
"	Totamol (1)	CP Pharmaceuticals.	"	Probeta LA (1)	Trinity
Betaxolol	Kerlone (1)	Lorex	"	Propanix (2)	Ashbourne
Bisopropol	Emcor (1)	Merck	Sotolol	Beta-cardone (1)	Evans
"	Monocor (1)	Wyeth	"	Sotacor (1)	Bristol-Meyers
"	Monozide (2)	Wyeth	Timolol	Betim (1)	Leo
Celoprolol	Celectol (1)	Rhone-Poulenc Rorer	"	Blocadren (1)	Merck Sharp & Dohme
Esmolol	Brevibloc (1)	Sanofi Winthrop	"	Moducren (2)	Merck Sharp & Dohme
Metoprolol	Betaloc (1)	Astra	"	Prestim (2)	Leo
"	Co-Betaloc (2)	Astra	§ Figures in parentheses indicate number of active ingredients		
"	Lopressor (1)	Geigy	§ Unbranded (generic) products not included		
Nadolol	Corgard (1)	Sanofi Winthrop	§ Drugs with alpha and beta blocking action not included		
"	Corgaretic 40 (2)	Sanofi Winthrop			

Table II. Further Examples of proliferation of drugs

Approved Name	Brand Name	Drug Comany	Approved Name	Brand Name	Drug Comany
H2 Antagonists for Peptic Ulcer.			Calcium Chanel Blockers for Angina, hypertension		
Cimetidine	Algitec (2)	SmithKlein Beecham	Amlodipine	Istin (1)	Pfizer
"	Dyspament (1)	SmithKlein Beecham	Diltiazem	Adizem XL (1)	Napp
"	Galenamet (1)	Galen	"	Angitil SR (1)	Trinity
"	Tagamet (1)	SmithKlein Beecham	"	Tildiem LA (1)	Lorex
"	Zita (1)	Eastern	"	Dilzem (1)	Elan
Famotidine	Pepsid (1)	Merck Sharp & Dohme	"	Slozem (1)	Merck
Nizatidine	Axid (1)	Lilly	"	Tildiem LA (1)	Lorex
"	Zinga (1)	Ashbourne	"	Viazem XL (1)	Du Pont
Ranitidine	Zantac (1)	Glaxo Wellcome	Felodipine	Plendil (1)	Astra
"	Pylorid (1)	Glaxo Wellcome	Isradipine	Prescal (1)	Ciba
ACE inhibitors for Heart Failure			Lacidipine	Motens (1)	Boehringer Ingelheim
Captopril	Acepril (1)	Ashbourne	Lercanidipine	Zanidip (1)	Napp
"	Acezide (2)	Ashbourne	Nicardipine	Cardene (1)	Yamanouchi
"	Capoten (1)	Squibb	"	Cardene SR(1)	Yamanouchi
"	Capozide (2)	Squibb	Nifedipine	Adalat LA (1)	Bayer
Cilazepril	Vascase (1)	Roche	"	Adipine MR (1)	Trinity
Enalapril	Innovace (1)	Merck Sharp & Dohme	"	Angiopine MR(1)	Ashbourne
"	Innozide (2)	Merck Sharp & Dohme	"	Beta Adelat (2)	Bayer
Fosinopril	Staril (1)	Squibb	"	Cardilate MR (1)	Baker Norton
Lisinopril	Carace (1)	du Pont	"	Coracten (1)	Evans
"	Carace Plus (2)	du Pont	"	Fortipine LA (1)	Goldshield
"	Zestoretic (2)	Zeneca	"	Slozem (1)	Merck
"	Zestril (1)	Zeneca	"	Tenif (2)	Zeneca
Moexipril	Perdix (1)	Schwartz	"	Tensipine MR (1)	Ethical General
Perindopril	Coversyl (1)	Servier	"	Unipine XL (1)	Ethical General
Quinapril	Accupro (1)	Parke-Davis	Nisoldipine	Syscor MR (1)	Bayer
"	Accuretic (2)	Parke-Davis	Verapamil	Cordilox (1)	Baker Norton
Ramipril	Tritace (1)	Hoechst	"	Cordilox 160 (1)	Baker Norton
Trandolapril	Gopten (1)	Knoll		Securon (1)	Knoll
"	Odrik (1)	Hoechst	"	Securon SR (1)	Knoll
"	Tarka (2)	Knoll	"	Tarka (1)	Knoll
§ Figures in parentheses indicate number of active ingredients § Unbranded (generic) products not included			"	Univer (1)	Elan

Council, the Department of Health, the Prescription Pricing Authority and the medical defence bodies. The only way to surmount potentially formidable obstacles was to take them head on and alone. My experience with committees had taught me that if people have to band together to beat the bureaucrats, the probability of winning is low and the chance of winning within the term of office of one chairman is usually zero. Battles are won by maverick generals not by committees.

Several times during the late Seventies I was invited to lunch at the House of Commons with the late David Ginsberg. David was a Labour MP who later "defected" to the Social Democrats; he was also a leading figure in the management of the market research firm, Intercontinental Medical Statistics (IMS). This company had been very helpful to me in my work on the pill. Without their estimates for sales I would not have been able to make the comparisons between the various versions of the pill and the reports of thrombosis that led directly to the much safer mini pill. David said he regarded me as the leader in the field of adverse reactions monitoring. He planned to set up a medical department and wanted me to head it. I much enjoyed our lunches together and the opportunity to meet his parliamentary colleagues from both sides of the House, but I declined the kind offer because I believed that monitoring of patients should not be done through contracts with commercial organisations.

I decided to produce a textbook, collecting the world's best opinions and experience to use as a framework of scientific and administrative experience on which to build the institution I planned to set up. The task of assembling the book and getting fifty or more authors to submit their contributions on time was daunting and would have been quite impossible without the help of my wife, June. The plan for the book was simple. I drew a diagram based on a cart-wheel. The axle represented the patient, the hub represented her main sources of information, her general practitioner, her newspaper and her TV set. Arranged around the rim of the wheel and connected by the spokes were the other bodies contributing to all aspects of her health care. They included the Department of Health, hospital consultants, statisticians, epidemiologists, the drug industry, lawyers, pharmacists, consumer organisations and many others. I then approached representatives of each discipline and invited them to write about their current work and to discuss their relations with every other group shown on the diagram. The book was arranged in five parts, each linked by an introductory chapter by myself. The first edition of *Monitoring for Drug Safety* was published in 1980 in time for the open-ing of the Drug Surveillance Research Unit (DSRU) in Southampton. Sir John (later Lord) Butterfield wrote an excellent preface. One reviewer described it as not the only book on the subject but certainly the best. Fifty-nine men and three women from twelve countries had contributed to the work.[45]

For nearly two years John Butterfield, the Regius Professor of Physic in Cambridge, negotiated on my behalf in the hope of locating the new unit in Cambridge. A possible site was at the new Addenbrooke's Hospital recently built to the south of the City. I had begun to look forward to working alongside old colleagues and friends in Cambridge. One stum-bling block, however, was that my project would have to be agreeable to the incoming Professor of Clinical Pharmacology, and as nobody had yet been identified who could fill this post, John warned me long delays were likely. The notion that a major national project for post-marketing sur-veillance in general practice should depend on the appointment of a uni-versity pharmacologist was a passport to disaster. Pharmacologists are low on the list of people who need to be involved in the design of GP monitoring schemes. Their role is to do high technology research into the mechanisms of drug activity and toxicity in the laboratory and in clini-cal departments and to teach people about the way drugs work. Unfortunately, civil servants with responsibility to promote measures for improving drug safety have wrongly assumed that pharmacologists rather than practising clinicians and especially general practitioners are the best people to appoint as advisers on post-marketing surveillance. This is encouraged by the drug industry which is dependent on departments of pharmacology to investigate its products. They have an interest in people who may be in an influential position. Pharmacologists in turn are dependent on contracts with the industry for a large part of the financial support required to run their departments. I recognised that any institution I might establish would also depend on the industry for support, but it would have to be non-contractual and without "strings" of any kind. I could see that dependence on a university department of pharmacology was not compatible with a purely general practice scheme.

I discussed the project with Donald Acheson, who was then the founder and first Dean of the medical school in Southampton and who later became the Chief Medical Officer at the Department of Health. There was no reason why the Unit should not become part of the Faculty of Medicine at the University of Southampton. No progress was made in Cambridge throughout 1978 and as I had already collected pledges of substantial funding I decided to focus on Southampton. It would have been very pleasant to work in Cambridge where I had dreams about a Fellowship at my own college, and perhaps some teaching duties at the medical school. After all, I was the first student to qualify from Addenbrooke's long before it became the centre for the medical school.

I had been promised significant support from the Chief Scientist's Office at the Department of Health and my salary as a Principal Medical Officer would be paid until I had raised enough money to cover all the costs. It was very obvious, however, that I would have to look to the pharmaceutical industry for the bulk of the funds. Safety monitoring had to be non-specific in the sense that we must be prepared to study any drug, irrespective of whether or not its manufacturer wished us to. It could not be done on a contract basis. I needed large charitable donations.

My plans were very much on the lines of the original Recorded Release idea but less complicated. It would be a signalling or early warning system raising hypotheses about potential hazards, but would never amount to (nor ever has been) more than a simple tool to identify and roughly measure the incidence of new problems and help us to decide if there was a need for sophisticated epidemiological studies.

I called the new scheme Prescription-Event Monitoring (PEM). Patients who had been prescribed particular drugs would be identified from their prescriptions. When a prescription is dispensed the pharmacist's costs have to be reimbursed. The prescription forms pass to the Prescription Pricing Authority (PPA), where a team of about two thousand clerks expertly price them and enter the details onto a computer. Nearly five hundred million prescriptions are processed each year in England (PEM does not cover Wales, Scotland or Northern Ireland). The total cost of the drugs prescribed is more than £4,000 million and each person receives, on average, about ten prescriptions costing, on average about £9 each. For PEM, it would be necessary for the PPA's clerks to set aside all the prescriptions for the new drugs we wished to monitor and then send photocopies to the monitoring centre. Shortly after I retired fourteen years later it had become possible to avoid the intermediate stages of photocopying and processing tens of thousands of pieces of paper. The data were transferred directly from the PPA's computer to ours without any intermediate coding. Each prescription uniquely links a doctor and a patient with one or more drugs; it was the first essential component of PEM. The second component, the details of the events that followed taking the drug, would have to be extracted from the patient's medical records by the doctor who wrote the prescription.

The patients would be studied under the conditions of normal day-to-day medical practice rather than the artificial conditions of clinical trials.

In clinical trials it is usual to exclude certain groups of patients such as children, women of child-bearing age, frail or elderly patients or those who are seriously ill. They may be unduly sensitive to drugs and react badly but their exclusion may lead to the belief that a drug is safer than it really is. The majority of new drugs turn out to have a low and acceptable incidence of side-effects. Occasionally, however, an unexpected hazard emerges and when it does, the sooner its importance is assessed the better. By capturing most of the "events" occurring in a population of patients of known size, it should be possible to estimate the size of risks in a way that has always been impossible with yellow cards.

My case for sponsorship was based on the credibility of research not directly paid for by a drug company. My presentations to the industry and to the bodies approving PEM were identical. The main aims would be to confirm safety under real-life conditions, to detect previously unexpected hazards and determine how often they occurred. I emphasised that the Unit must be seen to be independent and not a contracting organisation. The Unit, and not the manufacturers, would choose which drugs or which problems would be studied. The method would be standardised so that the results with one drug could be compared with other similar drugs. The results of every study, good or bad, would be published.

Top priority would be given to keeping GPs informed of our interpretation of the data they had provided. This was essential for the safety of their patients or it would not be possible to retain their co-operation. Because of the uncertainty of acceptance and delays in the publication of conventional papers in widely read medical journals, it would be essential for the Unit to distribute its results to all GPs rapidly, probably in some form of house journal. We would share all the results with the manufacturer, irrespective of whether they had contributed to the Unit's funds, but they would not own the intellectual rights to the data. We would also circulate all the results to the international regulatory agencies.

Because a seemingly innocent "me too" drug might be the one that produced the next major hazard we would attempt to include them all in the screening process. We recognised, however, that with some large groups (heart drugs, NSAIDs, tranquillisers and antibiotics) there were so many new introductions that it would probably be impossible to include all of them. In deciding priorities we might have to take account of experience gained in other countries where the drug had been marketed earlier than in the UK. The information from PEM is available to any legitimate user. Data sent to the Medicines Control Agency by drug companies is not widely available because it is classed as "commercial in confidence." This lack of transparency would never be allowed to obscure information collected by the new Unit. Most company medical departments decided that the advantages of being seen to be independent outweighed the advantages of company exclusivity.

In 1979, I was joined by Dr. Kenneth Carter, an English doctor who was about to retire from the Syntex Corporation in Palo Alto, California. He had been a delegate at the Honolulu conference at which I presented my ideas and he made a considerable contribution to kick-starting the venture. Ken was doubly qualified in pharmacy and medicine and he had an encyclopaedic knowledge of the industry which proved invaluable in my early quest for funds. Not surprisingly, our first approach was to his former employers. We visited Syntex in Palo Alto and secured a promise of a six-figure grant, spread over five years, with no "strings." Other similar pledges followed and in December I was sufficiently confident in the financial backing for the project to take the proposal back to Southampton. I met with Donald Acheson, Jack Howell, the new Dean of Medicine who was to succeed him, and Charles George, Professor of Pharmacology. I highlighted the main objectives. The first was to set up PEM on a national scale as already described. The second was to provide facilities for ad hoc problem-solving studies using methods similar to those I had already tried with some success while working for the CSM. The third objective would be to collaborate with other specialist centres in setting up teaching programmes. Donald Acheson and his colleagues agreed the Unit could become part of the Faculty of Medicine at Southampton University.

On December 12th 1979, the University Senate approved the establishment of the Unit, subject to confirmation that I would be able to raise the funds. The University would be prepared to rent accommodation and would expect a substantial percentage of the funds for administrative services. Several companies had offered very large sums and one had even offered to sponsor the whole project. However, to avoid any risk that the Unit might seem to favour one or other manufacturer, I decided to impose an annual limit of £20,000 on the contribution from any one company. This restriction turned out to be good for credibility but not so good when I had to meet escalating needs for additional staff later on. Over the next fifteen years I raised over £9 million in "no strings" support from various sources. I succeeded in doing this without signing a single contract or agreeing to any restrictions imposed by drug companies or the Department on the use made of the funds or the data we obtained. I would have abandoned the project rather than stray from this path. An advisory committee was set up under the Chairmanship of Sir Ronald Gibson, a prominent Winchester GP and former Chairman of the Council of the BMA, to report progress to the University and the Department.

Nineteen Seventy-nine was another year of journeys, including a second circumnavigation of the world. In April, June and I flew to Delhi where I had meetings with the Chief Medical Officer, Dr. Ghotoska, and the head of the Indian Medical Research Council, Dr. Ramalingaswami, both of whom were interested in the possibility of introducing some simple drug monitoring measures in India. The Indian Government was considering a plan to train "barefoot doctors" (often a village headman) who would be able to make simple diagnoses and deliver treatment. They believed they could become sufficiently skilled to decide if a sick villager should be moved to hospital and to dispense drugs for common conditions. They wanted to train one of these "paramedics" for roughly every one thousand of the population, no mean task when the projection for year 2000 is one thousand million! They wondered if they should consider some form of scheme for these paramedics to collect information about adverse reactions. I suggested that any scheme for collecting data on adverse reactions should focus attention on drugs used to treat conditions common in India, such as malaria and tuberculosis, rather than dissipate resources on the study of drugs for which information could be provided by WHO.

After the DSRU opened in 1980, I was distressed to discover that WHO policy prevented their International Centre in Sweden from collecting information from independent centres. They could only accept our data second-hand from the Department of Health, and the Department officials usually showed little interest in the data on new drugs that we sent to them, probably because their management at that time favoured support for PMS conducted directly by drug companies. I had promised the Indians we would never hesitate to pass on any information they requested about drugs studied in the DSRU.

We flew to Japan where I shared the platform for several sessions with Professor Takemune Soda, Chairman of the Organising Committee of the Kyoto International Conference Against Drug-Induced Sufferings (KICADIS). As in Honolulu the main topics had been subacute myelo-optico-neuropathy (SMON) and more general aspects of drug surveillance. As well as my platform duties I presented two papers on monitoring. I chaired the final plenary session and was set the task of summarising the conference. There was overwhelming evidence that many cases of SMON had been caused by clioquinol used as a treatment for diarrhoea and that many patients, especially in Japan, had suffered irreversible nerve damage. KICADIS was quite atypical of any scientific conference I had ever attended. A number of victims of SMON sat silently in the front row of the auditorium throughout the sessions together with relatives carrying photographs of deceased victims decorated with black ribbon. That one of the two co-chairmen was a non-Japanese in a wheelchair may have helped defuse a potentially dangerous situation. There had been street demonstrations against the drug industry during the conference and we felt somewhat uneasy about warnings that violence might spread into the conference centre.

There was some doubt about how many of the 30,000 alleged Japanese cases were of SMON or of other diseases of the central nervous system such as multiple sclerosis or polio, or diseases caused by environmental pollutants such as mercury in fish. There was genuine uncertainty about the reasons why the industry had not cut its losses and removed the drugs from the market. I had noted en route to Kyoto that the chief suspect, clioquinol, was still available in India and Hong Kong. It seemed to me that taking the drugs off the market might be seen as an admission of guilt. The fear of litigation could have been counter-productive, perpetuating the exposure of patients to an avoidable risk. It was unclear why, apart from isolated cases in Europe and Australasia, the epidemic had almost exclusively affected the Japanese, since the drugs were heavily promoted and used world-wide. I believed it was largely because in the West we tended to use clioquinol during short exposures to the risk of "traveller's diarrhoea", while the Japanese had been using large quantities for long periods. In my summing up of the conference I tried to bring the various groups of adversaries together:

> "Rather than argue endlessly about the causes of SMON it seems to me to be more important to ask ourselves what we are

going to do about other people with disabilities, whether drug-induced or not. Some of the Japanese SMON cases did not take clioquinol, so it seems that the drug is not the cause of all the problems. These people need just as much help. I have spent about sixty percent of my life in a wheelchair. I try not to identify with disability except when it suits! I do know that most disabled people come to accept their misfortune with dignity and almost always with humour. I am pleased to see that our disabled colleagues who are present today have retained both their dignity and their humour."[46]

This went down especially well in the front row. For the first time in five days I could see some of the SMON victims exchanging knowing looks and even smiles.

After KICADIS, June and I flew from Osaka to Tokyo to discuss the Japanese translation of my book and then to San Francisco and home via New York. I returned to San Francisco in August, and thence to Portland, Oregon, for another conference and to Kalamazoo, Philadelphia and New York for more fund-raising presentations. Eventually perhaps four-fifths of all the support for the Unit was to be from US companies. Ken Carter and his wife rented a house in Winchester so he could continue to help with the fund raising and setting up of the unit.

***

The Drug Surveillance Research Unit (DSRU) opened its doors in June 1980 in two rooms allocated to us. I recruited two secretaries, Frances Gibson and Susan Richards; a statistician, Nigel Rawson, who had worked on the national whooping cough study with Professor Miller in London, and a Senior Research Fellow, Dr. Lynda Wilton. Lynda joined the Unit in

January 1981 (and remains after seventeen years as the longest serving member of staff), and in the same month Keith Castle, who had
been one of my yellow card team at the Department, joined us to
supervise the young women, some of them school-leavers in their first
jobs, who processed the prescriptions and follow-up forms. Gill
Pearce, an information scientist, joined us to develop the Unit's computer section and a little later Marilyn Skipp replaced Keith Castle in
charge of the coding staff. Nigel was able to get his PhD on the early
development of the methodology and subsequently obtained a chair in
Saskatchewan, Canada. Lynda specialised in "follow-up," particularly
of reports of fatalities, and later headed what became known affectionately as the "Death Squad." Others joining us for varying periods
as staff or project researchers included Mr. Tom Lucas, Dr. Joan Clarke,
Dr. Chris Spiers, Dr. Patrick Waller, Prof. Walter Spitzer, Dr. Guy
Edwards, Dr. Jane Andrew and Dr. Kiyoshi Kubota, and several overseas graduate students, all of whom made valuable contributions to
the Unit's development.

My final task before launching PEM was to secure the co-operation
of GPs and I anticipated that my greatest hurdle would be to convince
the British Medical Association (BMA) that PEM would be workable
and ethical. Dr. John Ball, a general practitioner from Worcester,
played a crucial role. John was Chairman of the General Medical
Services Committee (GMSC) of the BMA whose support was essential. I
spoke for three quarters of an hour at a crucial meeting with the GMSC.

I promised that the work imposed on GPs would not be heavy. We
anticipated posting between fifty and one hundred thousand forms
each year, an average of perhaps four per GP per year. Prescribing
would not be uniform because many doctors are cautious about new
drugs, but it was hoped that even heavy prescribers would be unlikely
to be asked to complete more than one or two forms per month. Next

I had the delicate task of telling the Committee there would be no pay-ment for doctors. Even if we were able to raise the funds, any pay-ment would suggest we were trying to stimulate prescribing of a par-ticular drug and would damage our credibility. Our approach to each doctor would be delayed up to a year after he had prescribed for an individual patient. PEM could not introduce any user bias by influ-encing his prescribing. The greatest objection to company-sponsored PMS, is that the patient is not a fully informed volunteer when she is entered into a trial and the new drug is prescribed. There was no need for this in PEM because the patient would already have been treated long before we approached the doctor. Many patients could have com-pleted their treatment several months before contacting him.

Finally I came to the vital questions of confidentiality and consent. The DSRU's rules would be based on the recommendations of a spe-cial committee of the Medical Research Council on the Use of Medical Information in Research (UMIR).[47] Confidentiality would be absolute. No identities of doctor or patient would ever be revealed outside the Unit. At this point in my presentation John Ball interrupted me, saying I was being far too modest. He said that on no occasion during the last sixteen years had any doctor been in trouble or any patient harmed as a result of my handling tens of thousands of reports for the CSM. He regarded this as the strongest point in favour of support for PEM in Southampton. To my great surprise and relief all the members of the GMSC stood up and applauded. The meeting was over and I had their support. At lunch I was told that they had agreed to the proposal only because they trusted me to resist political and drug-company interference and that they would not have agreed if the DSRU was to have been run by the CSM or the Department!

Meanwhile in Newcastle, Eric Stabler, a senior executive of the Prescription Pricing Authority (PPA) and enthusiast for PEM, had convinced his colleagues that it would be possible to photocopy the prescriptions (providing I could cover the cost). The two essential components of Prescription-Event Monitoring had now been brought together. I had one more meeting with the Central Ethical Committee of the BMA to reassure them about the confidentiality safeguards and the way was now clear to start working the scheme.

During two years of consultation I had shared my ideas for PEM with many people, but I was not aware that a former colleague at ICI, the late Michael Mungavin, had set up a company known as Medical Monitoring and Research Ltd. and had come to some arrangement with the Royal College of General Practitioners to establish a Medicines Surveillance Centre. According to their press release on October 15th 1980, the intention was to provide "a full service to the pharmaceutical industry." I did not attend the launch or the press conference, but "spies" reported that much of the proposal seemed to be identical to my specification for Southampton University. The estimated cost of monitoring a drug in their scheme was at least five times that of PEM, presumably because they intended to pay a fee to the doctor for each patient treated and to make a profit for themselves. Their homework had not been as thorough as mine and the project foundered soon after it was launched. I doubt if they would ever have been granted access to prescriptions.

The full title of the new unit in Southampton was the "Post-Marketing Drug Surveillance Research Unit" which we later shortened to "DSRU." Some time after we had started, Intercontinental Medical Statistics Ltd (IMS) set up a "Postmarketing Drug Surveillance Unit" to do studies for the industry. The close similarity to the title of our unit raised a few wry smiles in Southampton University. In 1986, when the DSRU's status was changed to that of a charitable trust, we felt that the word "surveillance" was too emotive, conjuring up "Big Brother" images, so we swapped the word "safety" for "surveillance" and became the Drug Safety Research Unit while retaining the acronym "DSRU."

In our first studies we were helped by an old friend from my days in Kent, Bill Williams, who equipped us with a small number of stand-alone computers called "Superbrains." They had very limited capacity, and as soon as we could afford it were replaced by a more powerful International Computers Ltd (ICL) installation with linked visual display units (VDUs). Later still an even more sophisticated system of VDUs and personal computers was built around a large capacity IBM AS400 machine. The computers provided rapid links between hundreds of thousands of prescription forms and the information culled from the GP's reports, and enabled us to see important differences in the adverse event profiles in exactly the same way we had examined differences in the adverse reaction profiles in my days with the Committee on Safety of Drugs (CSD). Later we were joined by Dr. Kiyoshi Kubota who developed the analytical methodology to a high degree of sophistication, enabling the profiles of some forty different drugs studied up to that time to be compared and contrasted. Kiyoshi eventually obtained a Chair at the University of Tokyo where he is now working to introduce PEM into Japanese medical practice (already referred to as J-PEM). Kiyoshi's contribution to the development of PEM and particularly the methods for assessing the vast amounts of data on our computer was outstanding.

In the remarkably short period of six months, I had pulled off the greatest gamble of my life. I had founded the DSRU in order to conduct Prescription-Event Monitoring on a national scale. I had raised the funds, moved the family to Southampton, established an office at the University and recruited staff. All these steps had been taken without any certainty that my proposals would be acceptable to several bodies whose agreement was essential. There was no certainty that the

PPA would allow me to use prescriptions to identify doctors and patients and even less that the GPs would co-operate in sufficient numbers to make the scheme work.

9 The Opren Affair

Prescription-Event Monitoring (PEM) was launched in January 1981 from our small office in a house on the campus previously used as student accommodation. I held a press conference which the medical and pharmaceutical journals reported very fully. The "nationals" gave it a surprisingly good coverage, but one of them got its stories mixed and reported that I had said transplant donors were having their organs removed before they were dead! However, most of them got the story right and especially my warning about the damage often caused by premature publicity to drug risks.

On two successive weeks in April 1981, the *British Medical Journal* published "pump priming" articles designed to set the scene for our first trial run of PEM.[48] I also published several papers and book chapters to focus attention on what I called the "numbers game." It was important for doctors to understand the factors that determined the size of study required to detect problems at various levels of frequency. We were asking them to help us achieve a target of at least ten thousand patients in each PEM study. With this number of patients we could realistically expect to record a serious problem if it affected one or more patients in every three thousand who had been treated with the drug. Whether this event or a number of similar events turned out to be genuine adverse drug reactions and how important they were, would depend on subsequent enquiries about individual cases. The scheme would depend to a large extent on

GPs reliably recording most of the serious events they had seen, even if they did not believe a drug had been responsible. With more common events, for example those affecting one in every three hundred patients, we would expect to be able to make a reasonable estimate of the true frequency of the event.

The risk that may be taken when treating a patient increases in step with the severity of the illness. For example, we would certainly accept a moderate risk that a drug might kill a patient with terminal cancer if there was a chance of significantly prolonging survival or easing suffering. At the other extreme, however, we would not be prepared to accept a one-in-a-million risk of a fatal reaction to a cough medicine given to a child. Doctors' enthusiasm to participate tends to increase in step with the severity of the disease. They would co-operate in a study of a new stomach ulcer treatment that might replace surgery but they would be less likely to help with a treatment for hay-fever. Paradoxically, studies designed to detect and measure large risks are comparatively easy to set up because they require only a relatively small number of patients.

As a preliminary exercise to identify any serious problems that might arise, my family GP, Dr. Robin Marsh, and his colleagues agreed to a small-scale exercise. To avoid any risk of bias, we hinted that the full-scale study would probably be on Glaxo's new ulcer treatment, Zantac. When we visited the practice, however, we revealed the real target drug was to be Opren. The patients' records were rapidly located and the pilot experiment revealed no unexpected problems. We believed that the speed of location of records would be decisive, and there seemed to be no major problems, provided GPs' co-operation could be secured.

Knowing that not all general practitioners are members of the British Medical Association and that many of those who receive the *British Medical Journal* do not read it immediately, if at all, I arranged to send reprints of the two pump priming articles to all general practitioners to ensure they were adequately briefed about PEM. The articles were accompanied by a letter saying that some of them would soon be receiving questionnaires (always referred to as "green forms" to distinguish them from the CSM's "yellow cards") asking for details about patients they had treated with Opren or Lederfen, two drugs recently introduced for the treatment of arthritis. It was essential that no GP should receive a request to complete a green form before he had been fully appraised of the scheme and especially of the precautions we would take to ensure confidentiality. Disaster struck almost immediately.

The questionnaires were prepared on the Drug Safety Research Unit's (DSRU) computer and posted in Southampton directly to the individual doctors. They were posted several days after the date we had fixed for the mass mailing of explanatory documents that were the only means of informing all twenty-three thousand GPs. These briefing documents had been packed and addressed by a mailing agency and delivered by road to a British Rail depot in central London to be transported by rail to postal centres throughout England on the appointed day. The arrangements had been made with great care but an unforeseen event occurred that nearly wrecked the scheme before it had got under way. There was a strike by the Association of Locomotive Engineers and Firemen (ASLEF) and the mailbags containing the reprints were held up at the main rail distribution point in London for several days. Meanwhile the green forms that had been posted in Southampton had taken a different route and reached the GPs before they knew anything about the scheme!

This was a catastrophic start to the first project of its kind ever to be attempted on a national scale. Green forms were arriving in the mail of thousands of doctors who between them had treated a total of fifteen thousand patients with Opren and a rather smaller number with the less often prescribed drug Lederfen. Many of them were angry and it is possible some have had nothing to do with PEM since. The speed with which a new hazard can be detected and measured depends on the speed with which all the early users of a new drug can be identified and studied. This is why it is essential that a single institution should conduct PEM or a similar scheme immediately after a new drug is marketed. There should be no competition from commercially organised promotional schemes that would reduce the number of responses to that centre. If two centres had equal shares of the available information, the time to detect a hazard could be doubled.

The DSRU could not afford the £6,000 it would cost to post an apology to all the doctors individually so I wrote immediately to the medical journals, although I knew many GPs would not read my letter in them. The strike slowed our detection of what turned out to be a serious problem that was responsible for a number of deaths. Within three months it became apparent that Opren (known as Oraflex in North America) was producing a serious problem – jaundice – from which some patients died. Later there were to be a number of accusations that the DSRU had missed this problem. In reality and in spite of the delay caused by the strike, jaundice in elderly patients was signalled very clearly by PEM even though the number of green forms returned was much smaller than we had hoped for.

Opren and Lederfen, or to give them their official non-proprietary names, benoxaprofen and fenbufen (I shall refer to them by their shorter brand names since this book is for the general reader), were two examples of a large group of drugs used to treat arthritis and other painful conditions. They may be conveniently described by their acronym NSAIDs. This stands for non-steroidal anti-inflammatory drugs. This distinguishes them from the steroids which are very powerful synthetic hormones that may be needed in very serious conditions such as rheumatoid arthritis. More than twenty new NSAIDs had been marketed in the United Kingdom within the lifetime of the Committee on Safety of Drugs and its successor, the Committee on Safety of Medicines, and nearly half of these have been included in DSRU studies. All of them produce side-effects of one kind or another, the most frequent and worrying being that they occasionally erode the lining of the gut and cause bleeding which can be fatal. Unfortunately, elderly patients are at greatest risk of these complications and they are the group most in need of NSAIDs since the frequency of arthritis increases steeply with advancing years.

As far as possible, all PEM studies are carried out in the same way so that comparisons can be made between the pattern and frequency of events during and after treatment. We were unable to find important differences in the frequency of gut bleeding in very large groups of patients surveyed over the years. I believe there was little to choose between the NSAIDs in spite of the claims that each new one was less irritant to the stomach than its predecessors. It would not be appropriate in this book to discuss the scientific basis for believing that Opren might be more effective, but it had certain properties not seen with earlier NSAIDs that led some experts to expect an unusually good response in rheumatoid arthritis, the less common but more disabling of the two common forms of arthritis. In pre-marketing trials, Opren had produced two types of adverse reaction that had not been a problem with earlier NSAIDs. It should have made the authorities very cautious about releasing it for widespread use. Many patients developed sensitivity to light (photosensitivity) and some developed a condition in which the nails soften and tend to separate from the nail-bed (onycholysis). I had deliberately chosen Opren for our first experiment because the photosensitivity and the nail problems were so frequent and so well known before it was marketed. This would test the sensitivity of the new method. If we failed to detect these common effects and to estimate their frequency accurately, we would have to think again about the method. Opren was marketed by Lilly and seemed likely to "take off" rapidly. We expected to collect a large number of prescriptions and identify the patients quite rapidly. We had posted fifteen thousand questionnaires at the beginning of January 1982; this covered most of the patients who had started Opren immediately after its launch towards the end of 1980. I had hoped that at least twelve thousand would be returned. Because of the rail strike, however, only six thousand forms were returned but among these were eight cases of jaundice. This was a strong signal which was quite sufficient to need more detailed investigation to confirm that the jaundice had been caused by the drug. Eight cases that had not yet been confirmed by follow-up fell far short of what would be required to justify any public statement at this stage. We urgently needed to expand the study considerably. We reported our early findings to the CSM and I was in the United States talking to the manufacturers in Indianapolis when the UK media forced the authorities to take action.

I did not know at that stage there had been some disagreement about Lilly's interpretation of studies designed to show how Opren was eliminated from the body. This was a specially important consideration in the elderly who tend to excrete drugs or their breakdown products more slowly than younger patients. I left Indianapolis with the uncomfortable feeling that some of the senior management had seemed rather too dismissive of the DSRU's provisional results. The US attitude contrasted with that of Lilly's Medical Director in the UK who had shown more concern, certainly in his conversations with me.

Politically it would have been better for the DSRU if I had given these few jaundice cases more publicity before the authorities acted. However, I believe in a policy of restraint until field investigations have confirmed that a drug really is the cause of suspected adverse reactions whether detected either by PEM or the yellow card system. Both schemes provide valuable early warning signals, but these signals must be regarded as "internal" and not for general publication until the reports have been confirmed. It is all too easy to base official action merely on the numbers of events that have been reported. This can be a fundamental mistake because so often in drug safety work we find that many of the reported events are disease-related rather than drug-related. They are complications of the disease being treated rather than the drug used to treat it. Some events may be caused by concurrent diseases unrelated to the one being treated with the suspect drug. It is also possible they may have been caused by other drugs taken at the same time as the one suspected. No amount of fancy statistical analysis could substitute for thorough investigation of the individual cases with the alleged "Opren-jaundice" diagnoses. No realistic estimates of incidence could be made until causes of jaundice, such as gallstones, had been excluded.

Events were moving very rapidly and it would have helped if the CSM had been more approachable. The DSRU was often cold-shouldered by the Licensing Authority who seemed to resent our independence and success in setting up the second national scheme beyond the control of the Licensing Authority. The Licensing Authority and the Medicines Control Agency that replaced it might have been expected to be supportive of the DSRU but several influential senior staff were soon to move into posts in which they would become involved with commercially managed studies.

The yellow card scheme was potentially able to signal previously unrecognised problems and was available as a monitoring tool for any drug at any time, but it could not measure the incidence of reactions and suffered from gross under-reporting of events. PEM could only be applied to a few drugs at a time, but could measure frequency and give a more detailed picture of any problem that emerged. The two methods were complementary and both should have been run together under one non-governmental roof. I take some pride in the fact that I had been largely responsible for developing the first and entirely responsible for the second of the two national systems.

In April and May 1982, small numbers of stories about elderly patients with jaundice started to appear in the medical press. The collection of patients in our PEM study was stepped up and it was eventually expanded to include twenty-four thousand patients, among whom we found fifty-four cases of liver or kidney damage. Many of these turned out to have nothing to do with Opren. There were cases of gall-stones, cancer of the pancreas, and virus infections of the liver, all of which cause jaundice. When occurring in patients who happened also to be taking Opren, doctors, stimulated by adverse publicity, tended to blame the drug before their patients had been thoroughly investigated. Some patients had stopped taking Opren many months before they developed jaundice. Our study picked up only three cases of jaundice that had also been reported to the CSM. Follow-up showed that two of these three, who presumably had not been followed up by the CSM, had cancer of the pancreas! Finding so many cases of jaundice that could not have been caused by Opren emphasised the invariable necessity for follow up before making public statements about cases reported to the CSM or DSRU. At the close of our study, which was completed after the drug had been withdrawn in a blaze of publicity, we concluded that at most twelve of the fifty-four cases of jaundice had probably or possibly been caused by Opren. There were twenty-four thousand patients in the study so these twelve represented, at most, an incidence of about one case in two thousand. Five of the twelve had died, giving a possible incidence of fatalities of about one in five thousand. It was a considerably greater incidence than had been reported for any other NSAID and most people would regard this as sensible grounds for a ban on the use of the drug. However, at first, I had favoured less drastic action.

There can be no argument that Opren caused the deaths of a small number of elderly patients. The immediate cause of most of the deaths was liver failure due to accumulation of Opren in the body. The kidneys of a healthy elderly person are usually able to remove the body's waste-products as well as most drugs or substances derived from them. In old age, however, or if the kidneys are diseased, they may fail to remove drugs fast enough. The drugs accumulate and damage other organs, particularly the liver. One simple explanation that could have accounted for many of the cases was that the recommended dose of Opren was too large for elderly patients.

The recommended daily dose of Opren was two 300mg tablets. For elderly patients, however, one tablet, or even dosing on alternate days, would have been quite adequate. It would have been easy to manufacture a half-strength (150mg.) tablet especially for them. Rather than withdraw Opren it might have been sufficient merely to warn doctors about the risks of overdosing elderly patients and advising against prescribing it for those with damaged kidneys. General practitioners who prescribed Opren soon learned that the main practical drawback was the photosensitivity but many patients were prepared to tolerate it because of the pain relief they were getting. The late Dennis Potter, the playwright, who suffered for much of his life from a crippling form of arthritis associated with severe psoriasis, complained bitterly that he and many other patients were "left high and dry" when the drug they were relying on was removed. He was suffering from cancer of the pancreas and was visibly jaundiced when he bravely gave a long television interview shortly before he died. After Opren was withdrawn, several elderly patients complained to me that they were perfectly happy to wear a hat and cover their arms while enjoying their gardens. Perhaps the patients and their doctors were wrong about the extent of the benefit but was it necessary to ban the drug?

In the *Side Effects of Drugs Essay* for 1985 I suggested that we had not yet learned all the lessons that could be learned from the Opren affair, nor did I believe the whole truth had been told by the various parties involved.[49] Before laying all the blame on the manufacturers, historians would do well to study any departmental files for 1980-85 which may survive. For example, that Opren was only slowly eliminated from the body was reported to the authorities by Lilly well before the drug was marketed and should have prompted more careful scrutiny of the levels of the drug in the body, especially in the elderly. The Licensing Authority seemed to have mishandled the affair in a crisis situation. We were amazed by their lack of communication with the DSRU. We had the largest collection of post-marketing data in the United Kingdom and PEM would enable us to estimate the incidence of jaundice which the yellow card scheme could not do. Our data were passed to them as soon as they became available and could have helped them to resist demands for instant action until our PEM study and their follow-up of case reports was completed. Another curious feature of the affair was that the authorities appeared not to have considered the studies which were presented at the 15th International Rheumatology Congress in Paris in June 1981, fourteen months before they were forced by media pressure to withdraw the licence. At the conference twenty-five papers had been presented of which fifteen had Lilly employees as authors or co-authors.[50] Several groups of investigators had measured the levels of the drug in the blood at various times after a dose and had shown how long it took for the kidneys to eliminate it. Some of them had deliberately made these measurements in elderly people. One expert, for example, concluded that Opren

> "... may have profound therapeutic implications and it may be sufficient to administer benoxaprofen to older patients less frequently or in lower doses with good therapeutic results"

He had predicted exactly what was to emerge the following year. Lilly executives may have tended to play down the early evidence from correspondence in the medical journals and the DSRU's study, but how could anybody accuse them of concealing vital evidence? Why was the Licensing Authority so insensitive to all this very relevant information, much of which had been published at the Paris Conference? I can only speculate, but a possible explanation might be that nobody from the Department had been sent to cover the conference. I cannot believe that Lilly, who sponsored the symposium, had not extended invitations to the Department of Health. It was a bona fide scientific meeting and none of the papers was promotional. I remembered, however, that shortly before I left the Department in 1980, I had been refused permission to speak at another conference on new drug monitoring methods on the grounds it was sponsored by a drug company. This seemed to be a strange new development because the conference was to be attended by several members of the Committee on Safety of Medicines. I was told it was now against Department policy for officials to attend such conferences if there was any question of company sponsorship. If this was true and this childish and paranoid ruling still applied after I had left the Department, it is hardly surprising that officials were caught unawares by Opren.

In October 1981, acting on the data presented at the Paris symposium in June the same year, the company proposed to the CSM that their "data sheet" (a document summarising the way a drug should be used and the precautions taken) should be modified to include a warning not to prescribe more than one tablet (300mg) each day to elderly or sick patients. I was told that in November 1981 the CSM's officials had turned down the suggestion! Instead they asked Lilly to do more experimental trials. If true, this was quite astonishing in view of the difficulty sometimes experienced by the authorities in persuading manufacturers to make changes that might interfere with sales. The modified data sheet recommending use of the lower dose in patients with impaired kidney function was not released until May 1982. Even then there was no strong recommendation about use of low doses in the elderly.

Predictably, when Opren was finally withdrawn in August 1982, the CSM was blamed for not removing the drug earlier and for the inadequacy of the monitoring arrangements. "Inadequacy" is hardly the right word; when I left the Department early in 1980 I was not replaced by an officer of similar rank or experience. Most of the doctors who had worked with me had also left through frustration, retirement or offers of better jobs. Gill Greenberg had moved to the Medical Research Council, Cliff Ruttle and Paul Dendy to other divisions of the Department, Roger Vaughan to a post in the United States, Alan Wilson and Peter Weber had joined the Association of the British Pharmaceutical Industry, and Keith Lovel and Derek Zutchi had retired. The team of nearly a hundred doctors I had recruited to conduct ad hoc follow-up in the field was no longer used. Without them it would have been virtually impossible to determine the role of Opren in the cases of jaundice reported to the CSM.

After the withdrawal the CSM's Chairman, Sir Abraham Goldberg, was fed to the wolves in a BBC *Panorama* programme. I recall a previous occasion when Derrick Dunlop had been asked to do a TV interview and I had deliberately ruined a "take." On this occasion Abe Goldberg fell into the trap of the "camera-off" trick and seemed to have been quite unsupported by his officials. Nobody had protected him against the trick that this particular programme is prone to. The camera and sound recording continues to run after the "victim" thinks it has been turned off. On this occasion Abe was made to look shifty and to ask "Was that a question? Are we still recording?" No doubt much of what he probably did record correctly was cut out. One doctor wrote to a GP journal:

"I was appalled by Dr. Goldberg's silence, gesticulation and coldness. The subject was Opren and he did not appear to have done his homework. The yellow card system is ludicrous, cumbersome and needs revision, otherwise we will see many more tragedies."

Although no longer speaking for the Department, I did my best to repair the damage in an interview published in the same journal a week later:

> "Although Dr. Inman said he thought the "Panorama" pro-gramme on Opren had undoubtedly wrongly damaged the Committee on Safety of Medicines, he also thinks the episode may have the effect of increasing yellow card reporting. "People may be shamed into doing so who never bothered before. The yellow cards are the best for picking up unusual effects."

I have given many interviews on television or film and know most of the tricks but it is worth warning the unwary when TV interviews are con-ducted using a single camera focused on the interviewee. The interview is conducted with occasional shots of the interviewer's back as he or she faces the interviewee. Then there is a "nods and winks" session during which the performers remain silent while the camera records snatches of head nodding to simulate careful attention which are inserted appropri-ately when the film is edited. Later the questions are repeated with the camera repositioned to face the interviewer. The interviewee may then leave the room for a cup of coffee, followed by a girl with a clipboard demanding a signature to a document which permits any or all of what was said to be screened (which I have often refused to sign). At this point the interviewer may accidentally or deliberately change the wording of the questions!

In one television interview I was asked, "Tell me, Dr. Inman, did your system spot the problem with Opren?" I explained that when the alarm went off we had eight cases of jaundice and were in the process of fol-lowing them up to confirm or refute the possibility that Opren might have been responsible. When the programme was screened a few days later, the question had become an accusation. "Tell me, Dr. Inman, Why didn't your system spot the problem with Opren?" My answer would have been the same for either of the questions, but several qualifying sentences had been clipped. Put the first way, my answer explained how we had acted responsibly, not risking a panic by rushing to the media as soon as we had the initial reports. Put the second way, my answer sounded like an excuse for failure. I subsequently tape-recorded most of my interviews.

Shortly after Opren had been removed from the market, the yellow card system was severely damaged in an extraordinary action by the officials for which no reasons have ever been given. Because the identities of doctors and patients were not stored on the computer, the ability to retrieve individual case-records and to link reports from more than one doctor about the same patient depended on a Patient Index and a Doctor Index. Astonishingly, these essential card-indexes were shredded! My staff had created them over sixteen years and took pride in their ability to locate any report, together with all associated documents, within about thirty seconds without the help of a computer. An official at the Department courteously replied to my exasperated enquiry confirming these two indexes had indeed been shredded and wrote, "We do not now have a computer-aided check for duplication, but the medical assessors do weed out some duplicates when they meet together." There was no way the medical staff could check all the ten thousand-odd reports they received each year. Two essential elements of the yellow card scheme had been destroyed. Why had this been done? One can only speculate. Without the indexes, individual reports would be difficult or impossible to identify and link together or to follow up. When I complained to a member of the CSM, he was quite unaware these vital indexes had been destroyed! The phrase "cover-up" rises perilously close to the surface of the dark pool of obscurity surrounding the Opren affair.

Whether the damage can be repaired one can only guess, but the yellow card system is no longer in the forefront of safety assurance that characterised the Sixties and Seventies, even though the Department has at last provided the computer equipment we lacked for so long. Months pass without a single reference to it in the general practitioner journals that formerly carried stories almost every week, however unpopular these may have been among the manufacturers whose advertisements fund the journals. I was sad to see the yellow card scheme running out of steam after putting so much effort into developing it; but the sixteen years work and the sacrifices made by my family may be judged to have been worthwhile if only for my lucky discovery leading to the introduction of the safer contraceptive pill and a few other successes such as clarifying the halothane-jaundice problem.

In August 1982 I published the first in the DSRU's booklets in the series – *PEM News*. A local printer, Colin Strong, the proprietor of Hamble Valley Press and staunch friend of the DSRU for many years, produced a very high quality booklet of up to fifty pages for little more than fifty pence per copy. *PEM News* was unpopular with some manufacturers but was to become the essential channel of communication with general practitioners. It informed them of any problems that had been detected and reassured them when new drugs seemed to be problem-free. Although resources only ran to publication at roughly eighteen-month intervals, its concise style and lack of statistics appealed to busy doctors who needed to see their efforts were worthwhile and to grasp essential messages quickly. Some critics who complain about the lack of statistics forget that data which depend on doctors' records are usually incomplete and unsuitable for statistical analysis. Between starting PEM in 1981 and my retirement in 1994, besides eight editions of *PEM News* we published forty-two journal papers and twenty-four "Letters to Editors"; we circulated thirty-two technical reports to international government agencies and published fifteen monographs in another series known as *PEM Reports*. I also gave a considerable number of TV and radio interviews.

However, I still regarded this as a poor output that could have been considerably improved if we had been able to afford more medical and technical staff.

PEM News has also been criticised because the early publication of the results of the DSRU's studies, even in summary form, may prejudice the acceptance of papers for subsequent publication in scientific journals. However, if one waited for such publications to be completed, circulated for "peer review," accepted by an editor and then published, three or four years could easily pass before they appeared. Two years after I retired I was still waiting for publication of one study I had completed three years before I retired! Although I was lucky never to have a paper on a matter of public interest such as the pill rejected by the *British Medical Journal* or *Lancet,* some of the papers submitted to lesser journals reporting that a drug was safe (and therefore not newsworthy) were rejected first time, even by small-circulation specialist journals. There would be little point in asking GPs to complete the DSRU's green forms if there was no fast means of feeding back results to them. The place for the DSRU's results and those of other monitoring centres is on the desks of the general practitioners who prescribe the drugs and not in obscure and little-read journals or the files of drug manufacturers. Most of the criticism of *PEM News* came from the drug industry and especially its trade organisation.

The extraordinary contrast between the massive publicity about the small risks of the pill and the lack of publicity after thousands of deaths linked with asthma inhalers helped me to appreciate the capricious nature of risk perception, and especially the difficulty in conveying meaningful information to patients or, for that matter, to their doctors. In 1983, I was invited to deliver a lecture at Wolfson College in Oxford as part of a series of public lectures on "Risk."[51] There were eight lectures. The first was by Sir Herman Bondi on risk perception, the second by Donald Broadbent on the psychology of risk, followed by mine on the risks of medical intervention. Later speakers covered industrial or environmental hazards, and risks in energy generation or biological research. Fortunately I had more than six months to prepare the one-hour lecture. I was helped by a friend and frequent visitor from California, John Urquhart, who with Klaus Heilmann, an ophthalmologist from Munich, had also been seeking improved ways of describing risk.

In spite of attrition through disease, accident, famine and war, our species has increased explosively, particularly in the twentieth century. The population of many countries has doubled in less than a century. It seems inevitable we will outgrow our resources and that the only alternative to disease, famine and war is contraception on a global scale. We live longer, enjoy a higher quality of life and, as I suggested at the beginning of my lecture, "we have more time to indulge in one of our favourite obsessions, which is worrying about risk."

Records have been kept in the UK from 1840 since which time infant mortality has fallen from one in seven to one in five hundred: annual mortality in children has been reduced twenty-fold: that of the young adults (excluding military and civilian deaths in wars) has fallen ten-fold. All this has produced a large increase in life expectancy. This enormous improvement in health has been achieved by greater affluence, better food and housing and by the conquest of diseases such as tuberculosis, syphilis and smallpox (the only disease believed to have been eradicated world-wide). Some of the extension of average life-span can be credited to the drug industry. Unfortunately, because of factors such as fast transportation and population mixing, AIDS or drug addiction and because many people are living to extreme old age where their resistance to infection begins to fail, some diseases such as tuberculosis are returning and new types of infection are being introduced, including those caused by antibiotic-resistant strains of bacteria bred in our own hospitals. In descending order of importance I believe the three main factors determining life-expectancy are smoking, being over-weight, and what your ancestors died of. The side-effects of the medicines we take are very far down the list.

There is a story about two retired Medical Officers of Health swapping reminiscences in a bar. One asked the other, "Tell me George, after all the life-time of effort you put into improving conditions in your region, did it do anything to the death rate?" "No" said George after a contemplative sip at his beer, — "it's still one per patient." You cannot save a life, you can only extend it. In risk assessment we are dealing with the rates with which certain events occur and the probabilities that they may lengthen or shorten life-expectancy. Probabilities are numbers and people not used to handling numbers may find them uncomfortable.

Lord Rothschild, in his Richard Dimbleby Lecture for 1978, made the much quoted observation that "comparisons, far from being odious, are the best antidote to panic."[52] When attempting to explain the risks of drug treatment, I try to use the rates or probabilities of familiar events such as motor accidents for comparison with drug risks. Most drugs are comparatively safe and the results of such comparisons are usually reassuring. We have somehow to get across to people the notion that a risk is nothing more than a probability that something bad will happen. The probability that you and I will die is 1.0 (i.e. one out of one). Some people would find it easier to express this as 100%. The distribution of the various risks affecting me is probably not the same as those affecting you because of differences in our age, occupation, habits such as eating, drinking or smoking, or the influence of underlying disease from which we may suffer such as obesity, diabetes or high blood pressure. Each of these risks can be represented by a figure such as 0.1 or 0.2 (i.e. 10% or 20%) that contributes to the sum of all the probabilities that we will die, adding up to 1.0 (100%). The probability that we will die before we reach the age of one hundred, however, is now very slightly less than 1.0, and it continues to diminish as an increasing number of us live long enough to receive a letter from the Queen congratulating us on reaching our hundredth birthday.

The risks of dying because of drug treatment are usually small fractions of one in a thousand and they pale into insignificance when compared with the risks of accident or disease. The statistics for violent or accidental deaths are particularly useful when reassuring patients about drug risks because they can see themselves playing the role of risk-taker, even though their perception may be distorted by – "it can't happen to me." For my lectures I made a slide headed "The risk of doing something or being somebody." It showed, for example, that United States Presidents had a one in forty-five record of assassination, about the same as matadors whose annual risk was one in fifty-nine, per year. Only these two were at greater risk than a person who smokes twenty or more cigarettes each day whose annual risk of smoking-related death was one in two hundred. Company directors, rather surprisingly, were three times as likely to die in non-traffic accidents as coal-miners (1/550 and 1/1700 respectively). In the aftermath of the Opren affair, another anti-arthritis drug called Zomax was taken off the market in the US after a single death at a time when there were estimated to be two million users. The UK, with no deaths, followed suit.

Risks of medical intervention should be expressed as loss of life-expectancy rather than lives lost; it is not so much a question of lost life but of lost time. The loss of a patient who could reasonably expect to live for thirty years is perceived to be a greater loss than that of one who could only expect to live for five years. Possibly because I am old and fanatically "pro-life," I suggest that it is important to measure risk of death in relative terms as the percentage of residual useful life lost by exposure to any particular risk, including the risk of a medical or surgical treatment. Otherwise there is a danger the residual life-expectancy of an elderly person will be under-valued. Earlier, I gave the example of the effects of smoking in a young adult, who is only half as likely to reach seventy compared with a non-smoker of the same age. The risks must be calculated for the age-group in which a particular drug is most often pre-scribed. Sixteen years ago I said to the audience in Oxford:

> "Recent problems with anti-arthritic drugs have sharpened my concern about our perception of risk in the treatment of very elderly patients who have the shortest life expectancy and who are more likely to suffer adverse drug reactions than younger people. As I get older I think I might opt to trade some years for greater comfort and mobility. On the other hand, the less there is to go the more I want to hang on to what is left because there is such a lot still to do and it is such fun doing it."

Perception of risk depends not on statistics but on the extent to which each individual identifies with various types of risk taker. A young woman may worry about the tiny risks of the pill yet think nothing about hang-gliding. When all the passengers in a Boeing 747 are killed it is per-ceived as a disaster. When the same number die in separate car accidents, little notice is taken. If eight jumbo jets crashed in England in one week, some people might give up flying; but this is probably less than the weekly toll from smoking. As a born-again ex-smoker I successfully per-suaded the staff of the DSRU that there would be no smoking on the premises.

Arthritis may not be thought of as a killing disease, but if the conse-quences of immobility, the risks of joint surgery, drug-reactions and even depression and suicide due to prolonged pain are taken into considera-tion, there is an appreciable mortality. A diagnosis of the most crippling form, rheumatoid arthritis, could easily reduce residual life-expectancy by one third. Arthritis is particularly important when considering the safety of anti-arthritic drugs. If the risk of death from the disease is compared with the risk of death from treatment, no drug so far marketed has been too dangerous to use in rheumatoid arthritis, yet drugs have been banned which carried risks that were ten thousand times smaller than the risks of the disease. Withdrawal of a marketed drug is only justified if it is significantly more dangerous than alternative treatments which are equally effective. Even taking the highest estimates of the death-rate from Opren, the risk of using it was at least a hundred times less than the risk of the consequences of rheumatoid arthritis. It was a risk that many sufferers were prepared to accept. Following the Opren incident there was a spate of withdrawals of NSAIDs based on information of very dubious reliability.

As well as extending life-span, drugs have played an important role in the improvement of our quality of life. They can control pain, dilate the bronchial tubes and the coronary arteries and relieve the symptoms of many illnesses. One of the most important lessons I was taught as a young doctor by Leslie Cole and Laurence Martin was that the treatment must never be worse than the disease. Drugs may extend life but they may sometimes also extend misery. But who can assess quality of life, other than the patient? I once heard a clergyman, it might have been Ronald Knox, preaching on the subject of human happiness and suffering. He said something like this – take a bath, a bucket, a cup and a thimble and fill them all to the brim with water. When you have done this you will realise something very remarkable – they are all equally full!

I am sceptical of assessments of other people's "quality of life." As resources run out, some medical treatments may not be offered or some operations may not be performed if the patient is elderly, even though her quality of life might be improved for several years. It is easy for those closest to the patient to judge there is little or no residual quality of life.

Although they may not admit it, a "happy release" may spare them the task of looking after an elderly or difficult relative, hasten the realisation of their inheritance and stop it being whittled away in nursing expense. The doctor in charge should hear what the relatives say but should never delegate his responsibilities to them. We hear a lot of dangerous rubbish nowadays about euthanasia. A doctor who fails to relieve severe and intractable pain without excessively diminishing intellect is probably a bad doctor who should go on a training course at a hospice. Any doctor worth his salt is capable of managing terminal suffering and ensuring dignity when it is time to go. If he really believes that the way to treat his patient is to terminate life abruptly, he should have the guts to administer the lethal dose himself, like any other executioner, and not commit the ultimate act of cowardice by leaving the fatal act to the patient.

So what is the point of all this? I believe we may be moving into an era in which life-expectancy and quality of life may be reduced because resources will have to be rationed. A larger fraction of the earning power of the shrinking percentage of the population who are at work will have to be spent on looking after the elderly. Just as it may be seen to be anti-social to own two cars and clog up the roads, it may be seen to be anti-social to live too long and clog up hospital beds. There is one area, however, in which immense savings could still be made. I have already touched on it in earlier discussions about "me too" drugs and possible changes to the patent laws.

The risks of adverse reactions to drug treatment make only a small contribution to the threat to life-expectancy, whilst the benefits (efficacy) of drugs should make a substantial contribution to increasing both the quantity and the quality of residual life. Unfortunately, the present regulations do not ensure that the most effective drugs are always used. It is not a licensing requirement that a new drug must show more efficacy than existing drugs. If they were, enormous savings could be made in the drug bill and the money saved (I would suggest a figure of at least £2,000 million each year) could provide more nurses and hospital beds or research into treatment of conditions that are currently untreatable. Drug regulation and "pharmacovigilance" are focused on small dangers but largely ignore the benefits. The laws have evolved slowly over the years since thalidomide, but the pharmaceutical industry has had far too much influence.

The Medicines Act of 1968 had no impact on the vital question of whether most of the new and often more expensive "me too" drugs make any significant addition to the quality of life that could not be obtained with existing and often much less expensive remedies. My professional life has been spent on risk assessment and very little I could have done while developing both of the national monitoring schemes could have had much impact on the issue of drug efficacy. I have done my best to improve methods for measuring the first half of what I call the therapeutic equation that deals with risk, but the second half dealing with benefit remains virtually untouched.

Pre-marketing clinical trial procedures need drastic revision and regulations must be introduced to ensure that data on relative efficacy is available before licensing. The use of inert placebos to compare efficacy in clinical trials is questionable. Comparisons of efficacy should always be with the best available treatment. I would only volunteer for a trial involving a placebo if I had a very trivial condition. The most effective available treatment must always be used for comparison with the new product and if the latter fails to show an obvious margin of benefit, it should not receive a product licence for marketing. When a clinical trial certificate is granted it should specify very precisely how the trials should be conducted. The choice of drug used for comparison and its dose should not be made by the drug company. The Medicines Controls Agency should be in direct contact with the clinician who will be responsible for the trial. For thirty years the Act has forced the authorities to license drugs which have no proven margin of benefit yet sometimes turn out to have more dangerous side effects. However hard the industry may scream, revision of the Medicines Act to include assessments of relative efficacy as well as relative safety is long overdue.

Understanding the 'Therapeutic Equation" is essential for risk management. Very often it is impossible to complete the equation because essential information is defective or unavailable; nevertheless, a doctor is expected to make vital risk-management decisions — to treat or not to treat - to advise medical or surgical treatment - to go for a cure or to palliate? It is a complex business. He has to start with the individual's life expectancy and current quality of life and to decide how much risk he is prepared to take with treatments that might shorten expectancy rather than extend it or reduce quality rather than improve it. He may feel that his experience is sufficient to enable him to treat the patient himself or he may refer her to someone else. If he refers her to a specialist, he must still be prepared to help her interpret the specialist's opinion or to choose one of several options. If she settles on medical treatment, he knows that he cannot rely on personal knowledge of the relative benefits and relative risks of all the drugs available. There are simply too many of them; too little is known about their relative safety and almost nothing is known about their relative efficacy. Usually the GP will do well to prescribe the drug that has the best track record in his hands rather than 'try out' the latest remedy that has been advertised. If the response to established treatment has been poor, he may be guided by a specialist who has been able to assess the results of treatment with a new drug in large numbers of patients. The emphasis of this book and my life's work is unbalanced in the sense that I have been almost entirely concerned with attempts to improve safety. The drug industry has usually, though not invariably, supported me because serious accidents are rare and the risk to shareholders is usually small. Early recognition of hazards reduces the cost of litigation and confirmation of safety boosts sales. The greatest challenge for the next century will be to introduce measures for assessing relative efficacy so that therapeutic equations can be solved. Such measures will be vigorously opposed by the industry because it is often impossible to prove that one drug is more effective than another at the same level of risk or that one drug is safer than another at the same level of efficacy. The industry lobby succeeded in keeping consideration of relative efficacy out of safety legislation when it was introduced in the late Sixties and every company will oppose any new rules requiring them to prove margins of relative efficacy in comparison with their competitor's products.

10 Win a few, lose a few

In December 1984, while teaching in Bad Neuheim in Germany, I received a phone call to say that I had been honoured with a personal Chair at Southampton University. I believe this was probably the first Chair in "Pharmacoepidemiology" although other job specifications had been used outside the UK in the general field of drug epidemiology with equally meaningful titles. My title was rather a mouthful, but accurately reflected my attempts to apply epidemiological methods to the study of drug reactions. I am not a pharmacologist. Pharmacologists spend most of their time finding out how drugs work. I had spent most of mine trying to identify problems caused by their unexpected side-effects in general practice, rather than delving deeply into biochemical mechanisms. Pharmacologists' expertise is applied mainly in the laboratory, the hospital ward or in drug-company or university research. This distinction is important because some pharmacologists drawn into pharmacoepidemiology have been disillusioned because their scientific drive is blunted by the difficulty in reaching firm conclusions from the sketchy information extracted from general practice records. It is generally accepted by epidemiologists that the operation of the U.K. yellow card scheme or similar schemes in other countries is not part of epidemiology. This was obvious during my years with the CSM. Valuable though they were, the yellow cards could do no more than signal potential hazards. They could suggest problems but very rarely solve them. Only twice in sixteen years was I able to use the yellow cards in sophisticated studies. The first led to the mini-pill (chapter 2) and the second to settling the halothane jaundice problem (chapter 4). I did, however, use epidemiological methods in several studies of the pill in which the starting point was a patient's death certificate. A group of known size, for example women of child-bearing age who developed thrombosis during one year, could be assembled by the Registrar General's office. They could be investigated to confirm that the diagnosis was correct, what conditions might have predisposed them to thrombosis and what other factors, such as oral contraceptives were involved. A "control" group of patients of the same age and sex could be used for comparison using standard epidemiological methods.

I believe PEM can be regarded as an admittedly rather crude tool in drug-epidemiology. The groups at risk are defined by the prescriptions but there is always some doubt about the completeness of the doctor's records and the amount of information he has transferred to the green forms. One cannot be sure, for example, if the patient took the drug that had been prescribed! Bathroom cupboards are often full of unopened or half-used bottles of medicines. A patient may collect a prescription and try to please the doctor by saying all the tablets were taken when this was not quite true. The main purpose of PEM is not to produce elegant and scientifically admirable publications, but to raise hypotheses, often of an extremely tentative nature, by showing differences when the frequencies of events in populations treated with different drugs are compared. If PEM identifies a potentially important hazard, more sophisticated epidemiological studies are usually needed to investigate it further.

Early in 1983 Dr. Geoffrey Venning, Director of Research at Janssen Pharmaceuticals, published a series of articles in the *British Medical Journal* based on a survey by twenty physicians.[53] Ten were doctors working in international regulatory agencies and ten in independent institutions. Each of us was asked to list, without putting them in any special order, the ten most important drug-safety problems we thought had been identified since thalidomide. Not surprisingly nineteen of the twenty picked the practolol incident (chapter 5) and seventeen selected thrombosis with oral contraceptives (chapter 2). Geoffrey examined the fifteen most frequently cited drugs in more detail and attempted to find out how each of these problems had first become known, how long they had been on the market at the time, and how long before there was any official action. He concluded, rather surprisingly and incorrectly, that the CSM's yellow card system had failed to contribute to the first alert for any of the top fifteen problems. Although I was no longer responsible for the yellow card scheme, I defended it vigorously in a long letter to the journal, explaining why I believed his criticism was unfair.[54]

My main objection was that eleven of the fifteen drugs had been marketed before the yellow card system had even been started; one of them, phenacetin, had been available for seventy-seven years! Only three of the fifteen had been under surveillance by the Committee's yellow card system for the whole of their market life and the scheme was designed to detect problems with new drugs. Two of the three had revealed their hazards in reports to the CSM; this included an antibiotic called lincomycin. Its adverse effects were later described by the long-winded term, pseudomembranous colitis, a condition that was characterised by severe diarrhoea and bleeding, together with changes in the large bowel that could only be diagnosed after a specialist's examination with an instrument. The yellow cards had identified this problem one year after lincomycin had been marketed but we used the GP's description that in those days was haemorrhagic or bloody diarrhoea. The problem had been extensively discussed with the manufacturers and other national regulatory agencies but not given wide publicity. We had anticipated a similar problem would occur when the second of the three drugs, a closely related antibiotic called clindamycin, subsequently appeared on the market and this is exactly what happened. The apparent failure of the system in this case was simply because a new word was used for the first time to describe a collection of symptoms and signs already described in other terms. The use of new words to describe an old condition often credits its inventor with re-discovery of a condition that may well have been recognised by others under another name for many years. As an aside – the manufacturers of the first drug complained to the Chairman of the Committee that I had damaged the world market for lincomycin by consulting my counterparts in other countries to enquire if they had seen any similar cases! I was even reprimanded by a senior official for this entirely appropriate and responsible action - such is the influence of the drug companies. My response was probably not relayed to the company because it was unprintable.

Thus only one of the fifteen remained: the Eraldin accident (Chapter 5) had been missed completely by the yellow cards. However, the problem had been discussed with the Committee when the authors of the three papers that first drew attention to it informed us before publication. The Committee could hardly be blamed for deferring any action against Eraldin until these papers had been published The hole in the safety net was not due to intrinsic faults in the yellow card system; the adverse events had simply not been recognised for what they were and the majority of doctors did not report the many events which they must have seen.

In 1983, although the Drug Safety Research Unit (DSRU) was not yet working at full capacity, the monthly output of about ten thousand reports was already about the same as the annual number of yellow cards sent to the CSM. We rapidly outgrew the small office on the Southampton University campus, so I bought the other half of the old Georgian house where June and I were living and transferred the "Green Formers," the staff responsible for processing the doctors' reports, leaving the prescription-processing section in Southampton.

Our studies now included five anti-arthritis drugs, three of which - Opren, Zomax, and Osmosin - had been banned while we were still collecting prescriptions to identify the patients. Two others, Feldene and Lederfen, together with several more recently introduced NSAIDs have so far survived the post-Opren purge. Sixty-two thousand questionnaires had been returned and we had made a very interesting and potentially important discovery. It was of a possibly beneficial rather than a harmful effect. We found the rate at which patients suffered fatal or non-fatal coronary thrombosis attacks was greater after stopping any of these five drugs than while they were being used. For nearly all other kinds of event we had always found that the rate of reporting during treatment was higher for those patients who were still taking the drug than for those who had stopped using it. This was because doctors were less inclined to report events they thought were outside the period that would be of greatest interest to us. For most events the rate during treatment was fairly consistently forty per cent higher than after treatment had been stopped or an unrelated treatment substituted. For these five drugs, however, the rate of coronary thrombosis during treatment was only about half the rate reported after stopping it. This was very odd; there could only be two possible explanations for the larger rate after treatment with these NSAIDs had been stopped. Either there was some peculiar set of circumstances that had caused doctors to under-report coronary thrombosis occurring during treatment but not other kinds of event, or these five drugs were in some way protective against coronary thrombosis. Nobody was able to suggest why doctors should have recorded coronary thrombosis in this way, and this left only the possible cardio-protective hypothesis. It is now accepted that regular small doses of aspirin reduce the rate of heart attacks by interfering with the process of blood clotting. All the anti-arthritis drugs we had studied are likely to modify the same enzymes involved in the process of blood clotting.

There have been many arguments about the risk of using anti-arthritis drugs in the elderly, in whom bleeding from the gut is more likely to occur than in younger or more robust patients, but our studies had shown this particular risk was only slightly increased. I suggested to a number of people that the idea that the drugs might be protective against heart attacks should be tested under more rigid conditions. Unfortunately the withdrawal of six anti-arthritis drugs and the furore about Opren jaundice deterred potential investigators. It is easy to see they would not be keen to start a study that could take five or more years to complete if there was any risk of further withdrawals before their study was finished. As far as I know, no such trial has ever been attempted. We were careful to make no exaggerated claims and there was no publicity about our findings in the United Kingdom but in the US some newspapers asked how many Americans had died from avoidable heart attacks after these drugs were banned.

By 1985 PEM was accepted as a reliable method of post-marketing surveillance and it was expanding. There was a pressing need to appoint a Deputy who could take over from me in due course. However, there were serious obstacles and I had to battle on for a further nine years, coping with progressive weakness due to the "post-polio syndrome," the late effects of a whip-lash injury sustained in a rear-end "shunt" in my car, and life in an electric wheelchair, since I could no longer propel myself in a lightweight manual one. This greatly limited my ability to travel to represent the DSRU at scientific meetings and raise funds.

The number of potential candidates with suitable experience was very limited and many of them were employed in the pharmaceutical industry and earning at least twice my salary. The Director of the DSRU would have to be a full-time job and there was no chance that a senior doctor would be able to draw supplementary income from the NHS or private practice and at the same time run a Unit with more than fifty employees.

The University administrators insisted that, although the DSRU was entirely self-financing (I had raised all the funds), any departure from the normal salary structure would be resented by other people in the University. Even if this hurdle could be overcome in some way, there was an even worse restriction. The University would give no guarantee that anybody appointed as a Deputy could expect to take over my job when I retired. The job would have to go to open competition and the best performer in front of a large panel of interviewers appointed by the University would get the job. I could see no chance that anybody would be willing to join the Unit, move to Southampton and perhaps change children's schools as I had done, without a guarantee of succession. The solution to the problem was to set up a Charitable Trust and separate the DSRU from the University while retaining some sort of affiliation. A Board of Trustees was appointed that initially consisted of Sir Gordon Higginson (then Vice-Chancellor), Sir Douglas Black (a past President of the Royal College of Physicians), Prof. David Finney (the inspirer of event-monitoring), Dr. Dennis Burley (a leading pharmaceutical physician) and myself. The Drug Safety Research Trust took over responsibility for the DSRU on my 57th birthday, August 1st, 1986. Later the Trust was joined for a short period by Dr. Stephen Lock, a former Editor of the *British Medical Journal,* and later by Professor Stephen Holgate and Professor Charles George from Southampton University and my friend of thirty years, Professor Martin Vessey from Oxford.

Many people have asked how it has been possible to maintain scientific independence and credibility in spite of being funded by the industry. The policy that has enabled the DSRU to achieve this is quite straightforward. All the data from PEM studies, excluding information that identifies individual patients or doctors, are available to any member of the medical profession, the regulatory agencies, or research workers anywhere in the world. This is one of several features that distinguish PEM, the Unit's main source of data, from commercial post-marketing studies. If the latter show indifferent results, they are not published by the drug companies sponsoring them, their sole purpose being to encourage doctors to prescribe the product. Drug companies have absolutely no ownership or control over the intellectual rights to the data; they cannot delay or otherwise influence the publication of any results that might be commercially unfavourable. In many situations the company doctors were able to help the DSRU considerably with their knowledge of information gathered from their world markets. Of special importance was their ability to supply copies of everything ever published about their products.

Complete transparency, publication of all results and support "without strings," are the only ways to maintain the credibility of the DSRU. The choice of drugs or drug-safety problems to be included in routine PEM studies does not depend on whether the relevant manufacturer has agreed to cover the cost. The DSRU has not been deterred from embarking on PEM studies or from devoting resources to solving particular safety problems simply because a company is unwilling to co-operate. If a problem arises that demands an increase in the size or sophistication of a study, it may depend to some extent on obtaining additional support from the manufacturer and this was usually available. No contract, however, was ever signed in such a situation while I was Director. With few exceptions, the company doctors co-operated in an exemplary manner and it is difficult to see how we could have covered so much ground without their help.

The appointment of trustees raised the question often asked about members of the CSM or other similar bodies; should they hold paid consultancies with drug companies? The industry argues that if leading experts are not allowed to supplement their NHS or academic salaries in this way, the government would find it very difficult to get good people to serve on the committees. This may be true, but the dangers are considerable. As soon as they are appointed by Ministers, committee members are identified as people who are likely to have influence with government. They are offered consultancies to drug companies, ostensibly to advise them about their drugs, but in reality in the hope they may be sympathetic to any problem the company may meet in the future. Delmothe has shown that, in 1988, seventeen of the twenty-four members of the Medicines Commission, fourteen of the twenty-one members of the Committee on Safety of Medicines, twelve of the eighteen members of the Subcommittee on Safety, Efficacy and Adverse Reactions, and seven of the seventeen members of the Committee for the Review of Medicines, had personal interests in drug companies. Personal interests were defined as consultancies, accepting fees or share holding.[55] As far as I know, committee members are not paid an honorarium by the Government, merely their expenses, but some of them may hope to be rewarded with various orders of the non-existent British Empire or higher honours for what is often a major intrusion on their time and energy. If they really are *The Expert* in a particular subject, they may be the only member of a committee who possesses a particular expertise. As a consultant to the company, they have to "declare an interest" if that company's product comes up for discussion and it is not difficult to see that their elimination from the debate could be a considerable advantage to that company.

Over the years I have seen many examples of the way companies flaunt their "big names" to improve the company image, and sometimes even to advertise their products. The experts themselves often seem to be oblivious to the way they are being manipulated. It would be preferable if scientists serving on committees dealing with drug-safety problems were not retained by the drug industry. They should be free to give advice to companies on an ad hoc basis provided this advice is given openly. For example, they should be prepared to act as expert witnesses in court. Regular retainers, however, should disqualify them from service on government committees; it would be far better to pay them adequately out of public funds. We were very well aware of the fact that the staff of the DSRU have "insider information" and would be in a strong position to speculate on the stock market. Under threat of dismissal and legal action, no member of the staff of the DSRU is permitted to hold shares in any drug company or to pass information on to relatives or to anybody who might profit from it.

Since nobody can predict which new drug may turn out to be a "thalidomide" or an "Eraldin," the only safe policy is to examine all new chemical substances as they reach the market. The main limitation to the DSRU's ability to do this has been the capacity of the Prescription Pricing Authority (PPA) to supply copies of prescriptions and the willingness of GPs to fill in the green forms. Sometimes, if new drugs come on the market at a rate exceeding the PPA's limit, the DSRU has to choose those it considers most likely to prove troublesome. Many "me too" products seeking to capture a small piece of a lucrative market or to replace a drug that is patent-expired, are used to such a small extent that to include them would deflect resources from the investigation of more novel or more widely used products. A GP might do well to enquire whether a new drug he is thinking of prescribing will be included in the PEM pro-gramme. If not, or if the company says it is doing "PMS" itself (i.e. a pro-motional study), it would be safer to prescribe an established product instead. Several studies of drugs that failed to achieve a worthwhile volume of prescribing in a reasonable time had to be abandoned by the DSRU and we occasionally had to drop a routine study of a "me too" drug to make room for one that might be presenting a new hazard. The great-est blow to the Unit's image would be a major disaster with a drug that had not been put into the PEM screen. If such an accident occurred and the reason for omitting it from PEM had been the manufacturer's unwill-ingness to support the Unit, our reputation and credibility would be lost for ever. Several PEM studies have been done without the support of the manufacturer of the drug.

In the fourth edition of our GP booklet *PEM News* issued in March 1987, I summarised the principles that the DSRU would continue to operate under the management of the Drug Safety Research Trust.

> "The Trust will continue to work closely with the CSM, the manufacturers and independent institutions and to be supported by unconditional grants from many sources. Our primary tasks continue to be PEM of medicines containing new chemical entities and ad hoc testing of hypotheses generated either by PEM itself, by the CSM's yellow card scheme or by publications from elsewhere. Routine monitoring of individual drugs will be quite independent of whether their manufacturers are sponsors of the Unit. On the occasions that an important hazard has been detected which needs to be investigated in greater depth, we would expect the manufacturer concerned to provide additional funds in order to avoid draining the central funds contributed to by the other sponsors."

I continued to urge general practitioners to support both the yellow card scheme and the DSRU and referred to some disparaging press comments by the Department of Health, that were all the more surprising considering my spirited defence of their Chairman and repeated "plugs" for the system. I said:

> "I would like to stress yet again the need to support both national post-marketing surveillance systems – the yellow card scheme and PEM. The CSM's yellow card scheme continues to be the only effective means by which rare events, especially

those that are too rare to be picked up by PEM, can be detected early in the market life of a new drug. It is also the only scheme which is available for all drugs, new or old, all the time. I have been accused of running down the yellow card scheme or even of encouraging doctors not to use it. As the person who spent sixteen years of his life developing and managing the yellow card scheme for the CSM, it is hardly likely that I would wish to see it become extinct."

Since leaving the DHSS in 1980 there had been nine publications and twenty-two press interviews in which I stressed the need to support the yellow card scheme. It was true I had been critical of the Committee's failure to publish the evidence on which some drug withdrawals were based or to admit to the obvious limitations of any voluntary reporting system as a basis for scientific conclusions, but it was grossly unfair to accuse me of trying to undermine the system I had spent sixteen years developing.

In 1987, after meetings with Professor Bill Asscher, the Chairman of the Committee on Safety of Medicines, I devised a joint scheme we hoped might combine several advantages of the yellow cards and PEM. We called it the Red Alert scheme. Having identified the first ten thousand patients to receive a new drug with the help of the PPA, the DSRU and the CSM would amalgamate the information derived from the CSM's yellow cards and the DSRU's green forms. This would provide a better estimate of the incidence of events, and duplications would be avoided. The DSRU printed a special version of the CSM's Yellow card which carried a red triangle symbol. Unlike the normal cards, these "Red Alert" cards were addressed to the DSRU rather than the Committee and provided with sprocket holes at the margins so that they could be processed by our equipment. The idea was that we would "personalise" ten thousand yellow cards and send them to the doctor who had prescribed the new drug, asking him to keep them in each patient's record. He would use them only if he suspected an adverse reaction to the drug. After processing using the PEM routine, we would pass them to the CSM so they could also incorporate them in their normal yellow card procedure. Later, we would post green forms to all the doctors in the normal way and capture any information about important events that might not have been picked up by the Red Alert cards or the committee's yellow cards.

We applied the Red Alert scheme to four new drugs and at first it worked very well. It considerably increased the flow of yellow cards to the CSM and in all but one respect was problem-free. The scheme failed for a curious reason that neither Bill Asscher nor I had anticipated. The officials at the Licensing Authority decided they could not pass information to the DSRU about any yellow cards that had by-passed the new scheme and been reported directly to the Authority (even though they described adverse reactions in patients who had already been identified by the DSRU from prescriptions we had processed). It was important, for example, to include reports from doctors working in hospitals who are not sent green forms. They would report directly to the CSM on normal yellow cards and might be the first to see serious reactions in cases admitted to hospital. It was even possible a doctor might report to both the CSM and DSRU about the same patient at different times We were denied the means of combining the two sets of data and checking for duplications or missing data. We were in the almost unbelievable position of running a joint scheme which could have proved to be a great advance in drug safety monitoring when neither the Chairman of the CSM nor the Director of the DSRU, who were considered to be competent to manage the two national systems separately, was permitted to combine the data so a complete reaction profile of a drug could be constructed! The Red Alert scheme could have marked a turning point in the development of the national safety net. This incident reinforced my long-held view that the yellow card scheme should be separated from the Medicines Control Agency and run with PEM under the same roof or at least in parallel as a fully independent system, and not by civil servants. Like PEM it should operate in a non-political, non-commercial environment. This extraordinary ruling reflected the powerful influence of the manufacturers, who were determined to kill the scheme at all costs and on officials who supported drug company PMS. Certainly the manufacturers were delighted when the Red Alert scheme collapsed. They hated the idea that the name of any new drug should be associated with a red triangle, the traditional warning of danger. Historians will be interested in the files of this period.

In 1987 there was a further large expansion of the DSRU's staff. Our very popular General Manager, John Rogers, retired to work part-time as a teacher of English literature at the University's Department of Adult Education and Nigel Rawson obtained his PhD and moved to London before taking a Chair in Pharmacoepidemiology at the University of Saskatchewan. We were joined for about a year by Bill Cox, a Southampton businessman, to help the Trust raise funds. We decided to transfer the prescription processing section and the computer to offices above a shop in the nearby village of West End while we looked around for larger premises.

I have already described how, after devoting the most active sixteen years of my professional career to establishing the yellow card scheme and making it work, it was partially demolished by the shredding of the indexes in 1983. I had been only mildly surprised when the official recognition for my services to the community over sixteen years had been a short letter from a junior administrator (an "Executive Officer") who kindly wrote and thanked me on behalf of the Department of Health! PEM and the DSRU continued to be criticised by the Medicines Control Agency and the Association of the British Pharmaceutical Industry (ABPI). In spite of all their puff and blow, however, nobody has ever succeeded in getting an alternative nation-wide scheme off the ground. There were many bright ideas about how post-marketing surveillance should be done. Most of them played into the hands of the drug company sales departments eager to use PMS for promotional purposes. I had some supporters, however. In their report on the 1991-2 session, the Select Committee on the European Communities of the House of Lords said:

"We also received evidence of another system of pharmacovigilance in the United Kingdom, namely "Prescription Event Monitoring." It was set up by Professor William Inman initially at Southampton University Medical School and now has independent charitable status. The Prescription Pricing Authority supplies a copy of every prescription written for each new drug during an evaluation period of 2-3 years. About 10-12 drugs are selected for evaluation at a time and about 22,000 doctors are involved; they report on every "significant event" in the patient's experience while taking the drug. Once the data is transferred from questionnaire forms to a computer data bank it can be analysed by technically qualified assessors. A more detailed procedure is followed where patients have died during the study. The response is said to be over 70 per cent, and claimed to be much higher than the United Kingdom's yellow card system. Professor Inman estimates that his system costs about £150,000 per drug, modest when set against an estimated £80 million cost of the launch of a major new drug.

We recommend that the Commission considers the use of Prescription Event Monitoring throughout the Community. Its method of in-depth analysis of a carefully selected group of new products using data from a large random sample seems both effective and well adapted for Community policy."[56]

In 1988 I lost more "good conduct points" by producing some results that caused the MCA to lose an appeal in the High Court. At the time the MCA seemed to be ranging around for soft targets to reduce the NHS drug bill, a laudable enough endeavour but almost laughable when it produced the twisted logic that was involved. They had decided to remove the licence for a drug called mianserin that had been marketed for the treatment of depression by two companies as Bolvidon and Norval for nearly ten years. A small number of reports of blood disorders had accumulated over the years. As an alternative to another large group of drugs known as tricyclic antidepressants, mianserin had several advantages, being much safer for men with enlarged prostates who were at risk of acute urinary retention or for patients with a tendency to the blinding disease known as glaucoma. Even more important, their decision seemed to take no account of the vital fact that mianserin was a much safer drug if taken in suicidal overdose than these alternatives in use at the time.

I have already mentioned the serious defect in the Medicines Act of 1968 that precludes consideration of relative efficacy. Due to another defect in the Act, the MCA was not able to take the risk of suicide into account because it only permitted consideration of the *normal* use of drugs in the recommended doses. It excluded *abnormal* use by drug abusers as well as the consequences of accidental or deliberate overdose. The choices of treatment for depression includes drugs, various forms of psychotherapy, and even electric shocks to the brain or electro-convulsive therapy (ECT). The largest risk in depressive illness is suicide. At the height of their depression patients often overdose with the drugs most handy at the time – their antidepressants. Sometimes they overdose as an attention-seeking "suicidal gesture," believing the drug to be innocuous. Mianserin was often prescribed for elderly patients with terminal cancer

for whom the last thing wanted was the side-effects of the more powerful tricyclics.

I decided the DSRU should investigate the possibility that mianserin
might carry an unacceptable risk of blood disorders and I was encouraged
to do so by one of the Department's medical officers. We could identify
large numbers of patients who had used mianserin or any other drug we
might chose to use for comparison. The investigation would include suicides as well as blood disorders and I used a drug called amitriptyline for
comparison as it was the most frequently prescribed alternative. I asked
the Prescription Pricing Authority to send me photocopies of all the prescriptions for both drugs issued in January 1987. Since it was unlikely
many patients would receive more than one prescription during a single
month, each one should correspond with one patient. To my embarrassment, the PPA sent one hundred and eighty thousand prescriptions! I had
to cut the study down to a manageable size by using only the first six
legible prescriptions for each drug written by each doctor. The final
analysis was of twenty-seven thousand patients who had been treated
with mianserin and forty-two thousand who had been treated with
amitriptyline. This corresponded roughly to all the patients treated in
England during a period of only two weeks! In neither group did we find
any example of a severe or potentially fatal blood disorder. This did not
mean that the drugs were free from any risk but blood disorders were
obviously very uncommon.

Next I turned my attention to the "successful" suicides. Twenty-five
patients had used violent methods to kill themselves. Eight of these had
hanged, four had drowned, three "fell from a height," two died from knife
wounds, two from gas, two threw themselves under a moving vehicle and
the other four chose a shotgun, a corrosive fluid, a plastic bag and a can
of petrol respectively. Among those who survived a suicide attempt,
ninety had taken mianserin. Not one of them had required admission to

a hospital intensive care unit. Among two hundred and forty survivors of amitriptyline overdose, no fewer than fifty-six had been admitted to intensive care units! Among three hundred and ten survivors of attempts with other types of antidepressant drugs, seventeen had required intensive care. I estimated that in the country as a whole it was possible that as many as six thousand patients might attempt suicide with mianserin each year but hardly any would need intensive care or die. Similarly, up to fourteen thousand would use amitriptyline and nearly twelve hundred of them could need intensive care. This enormous difference could not be ignored, especially by those who were interested in the costs of hospital treatment. I concluded in the *Lancet*:

> "Clearly these negative findings do not exclude the possibility that mianserin may occasionally cause blood dyscrasias, as indeed may amitriptyline or other antidepressant drugs, but there is no doubt that mianserin is appreciably safer than many other drugs when taken in overdosage."[57]

The MCA contested my findings. They argued that safety in overdosage was not an important issue if there had been even a few deaths from blood disease. They also hinted that our results might have been favourable because the drug was being more safely prescribed at the time of my study thanks to the publicity given to their safety advice! If this was true, why had they suddenly decided to condemn a drug they had allowed to be sold for ten years?

The case against mianserin rested largely on unconfirmed hospital reports to the CSM. I was asked by the manufacturer to review copies of all the yellow cards sent to them with the names blanked out. I immediately noticed that many reports were from junior hospital doctors and that the date on the yellow card was quite frequently the same or within one or two days of the date of the hospital admission. There was therefore little chance that the doctor reporting the case could have had time to acquire essential details from the GP or the psychiatrists who had looked after the patient. Some cases could have been caused by the drug or by other drugs given concurrently, since multiple drug treatment is the rule rather than the exception in psychiatric illness. There were also several obvious duplicates, a legacy of the destruction of the CSM's indexes. This cast a shadow over the MCA's case against the drug.

The manufacturers appealed against the MCA's ruling to the Medicines Commission but their appeal was turned down. They then took the case to the High Court and on February 17th 1989, two judges, Lord Justice Glidewell and Mr. Justice Pill, ruled that I had shown very clearly that overdoses of mianserin were much less likely to be fatal than overdoses of many than other drugs and that safety in overdose was relevant. In the judges' opinion the Medicines Commission had been given incorrect legal advice. The Department continued to argue that they could only consider normal use of drugs. As far as I was concerned the Law Lords' ruling might be hard on the twenty year-old Medicines Act that tied the MCA's hands, but elderly patients who are depressed, perhaps because they are terminally ill, continue to benefit because the drug is still available. The MCA's officials had appeared to be pleased when the DSRU started the study, hoping no doubt it might add weight to their decision to remove it, but were not amused by the outcome. My problems with the MCA were not with individuals but with a system that puts them in a position in which they can profoundly influence public policy but which does not allow them ever to admit they might have been wrong.

Towards the end of the next story, colleagues were told by a petulant senior official that I had no business to be involved in a challenge to the MCA! She had forgotten, or was perhaps unaware, that I had been involved with this particular problem with a sleeping tablet called

Halcion while I was working for the CSM long before any of the present staff had joined the Department. My recommendations for the safer use of Halcion in 1989 were exactly the same as they had been ten years earlier when they were accepted by the CSM, long before the MCA existed.

Halcion is one of a large group of drugs called benzodiazepines, among which are familiar products such as Librium and Valium, the so-called "tranquillisers," and sleeping tablets such as Normison and Mogadon. Librium first appeared about 1960 and Valium two years later, rapidly becoming "cult" drugs that the "stressed" housewife would often find herself taking after visiting her GP. Mogadon appeared as a sleeping tablet about 1970 and rapidly established itself as a safe alternative to the barbiturates. "Safe" meant safe in overdose. Before the introduction of benzodiazepines, barbiturates were the drugs most frequently used by suicides. It was almost impossible to kill oneself with Mogadon. Halcion was introduced in 1979 and was generally thought to have a margin of advantage over all the others because it worked very rapidly and left little or no hangover.

In July 1979, the media in Holland reacted dramatically to what became known as the "van der Kroef Syndrome."[58] Dr. Cees van der Kroef, a much respected psychiatrist practising in The Hague, reported that he had treated eleven patients with Halcion; four had developed severe psychiatric symptoms such as aggression or elation, delusions of persecution or hallucinations not unlike a bad "trip" on LSD. He had reported his findings to the Dutch authorities who initially showed no surprise because they had already received a few similar reports. However, during a slack news week at the beginning of July, the page proofs of van der Kroef's paper mysteriously found their way to the media twenty-four hours before it was due for publication in the scientific press. What should have been a fairly low-key paper for doctors produced banner headlines and phone calls to the Netherlands Adverse Reactions Monitoring Centre from hundreds of alleged victims, some of whom undoubtedly had genuine symptoms. My friend and opposite number in Holland, Ronnie Meyboom, examined the evidence as quickly as he could and the licence for Halcion was suspended for six months.

In the United Kingdom, in spite of some publicity following the events in Holland, there had been only a small number of reports of similar complaints and I could find no evidence of a problem on anything approaching a scale resembling the "van der Kroef Syndrome" in Holland. In 1979 the CSM received twenty-two reports of mental side effects. Even if we made the assumption that perhaps only ten per cent of events had been reported, this was equivalent to about one case for every ten thousand prescriptions for Halcion. The doses prescribed in Holland were often four and sometimes eight or more times larger than those used in the UK and I advised the CSM that the most likely reason for the huge difference in reporting of psychiatric reactions in the two countries was simply the doses used. The Committee accepted this advice and decided that no further action was required.

In 1982, an article by Paul Foot in *The Mirror* produced a few reports to the CSM, but by that time the sales of Halcion had quadrupled, and the net reporting rate after this short-lived publicity was less than during the first two years of marketing. Thereafter the reports fell to four or five per year, and from 1987 to 1990 they corresponded to about one report for every one million prescriptions written by GPs.

In December 1991, twelve years after the van der Kroef incident, the MCA suddenly decided to revoke the licence for Halcion. This decision was astonishing since their case against the drug seemed to have been based almost entirely on alleged defects in the collection of data in a study conducted twenty years earlier in the United States. The Upjohn Company had commissioned a clinical trial in a US penitentiary in Jackson, Michigan, a maximum security institution for violent psychopathic criminals, including murderers. It is difficult to imagine a less suitable place to conduct a trial of a sleeping tablet, but in those days it was normal practice for pharmaceutical companies to commission trials in "volunteers" who could gain certain benefits by taking part in experiments with new drugs. The MCA's contention was that there were flaws in the data and the submission of the trial results had been unsatisfactory. They decided a licence should not have been granted. It seems incredible, however, that a defect in a study completed twenty years earlier could have any relevance to the safety of Halcion in 1991, without any new evidence to suggest the drug was unsafe. Moreover, after the van der Kroef incident, the drug had been reinstated in Holland and in most other countries, but the recommended doses had been reduced to one half or one quarter of the doses previously prescribed and were now the same as those used by patients in the UK.

The MCA's case against Halcion may have started as a piece of political kite-flying, perhaps part of a campaign to remove certain classes of drugs they deemed to be non-essential from the list of those which can be supplied by the National Health Service. They had found imperfections in a twenty year old clinical trial protocol and may have seen Halcion as a softer target than some more recently introduced sleeping tablets. There was no evidence Halcion was presenting any problems that had not been known for at least a decade.

The Upjohn Company appealed to the Medicine's Commission against the MCA's ruling and I was one of a group of people invited to help prepare the appeal. I was asked to review the yellow cards reporting alleged psychiatric reactions and it was immediately obvious that very few of them could be described as *serious* reactions. There had been a few reports of depression (which could lead to suicide) but many patients were sleepless because they were already depressed. The number of reports of mental disturbances was so low that virtually all drugs would have to be taken off the market if the same rate was applied generally. The DSRU's data for completely unrelated drugs provided some remarkable comparisons. "Aggression," for example, had been reported as a coincidental event many times more frequently in our study of a large group of patients treated with a drug for incontinence! "Depression" was much more common in patients treated with H_2-antagonists for dyspepsia. In short, the frequency of disturbances reported to the CSM as suspected adverse reactions to Halcion was considerably less than their "background" frequency in the general population. The MCA seemed not to have learned that spontaneous reports to the CSM or other similar bodies should never be used to calculate the incidence of adverse reactions. This is not to deny the value of the yellow card system but merely to reiterate its limitations. In their evidence to the Medicines Commission, several experts stressed that each report of an alleged psychiatric reaction to a drug should be assessed carefully by a trained psychiatrist. It required a degree of expertise that would be quite beyond what could reasonably be expected of the MCA's staff. The expert psychiatrists, among them Sir Martin Roth, emphasised the vital importance of discriminating between normal variations in mood or behaviour, and abnormalities amounting to a full blown psychiatric disorder of the kind reported in patients taking large doses in Holland. The MCA appeared not to have taken this important distinction into consideration.

The MCA also seemed to have ignored much of the history of the Department's involvement in Halcion and especially the views of the CSM in 1979. As part of the normal appeals procedure, a more experienced member of the MCA's own medical staff had been appointed by the Medicines Commission to reappraise the original paper. He came to the conclusion there was insufficient evidence from the adverse reaction reports to support the withdrawal of the product.

Professor Ian Hindmarch, the Head of the Psychopharmacology

Research Unit at the Robens Institute, had examined the drug for evidence of "hang-over" effects on mental function that might affect driving ability or occupations requiring concentration. Could taking a Halcion tablet at night cause an accident driving to work in the morning? Although a drug may delay a patient's reaction time by only a few hundredths of a second, as he put it – "this can make all the difference between stopping behind the car in front of you and stopping a couple of yards in front of it at the point where you would have stopped if you hadn't hit it first!' He had also studied experiments in air traffic control operators who work shifts involving frequent changes in sleep pattern. He had found no evidence to suggest Halcion had any peculiar properties that would make it more dangerous than other sleeping tablets.

A large delegation attended a hearing of the appeal by the Medicines Commission. For reasons never explained by the civil servants who stage-managed the meeting, we were subjected to the gross discourtesy of being kept waiting for four hours after the appointed time in a hot stuffy office without air conditioning while the Commission finished its business and then had their lunch. When we finally got to the meeting, several Commissioners shook hands or waved to me across the table but the civil servants pointedly avoided eye contact. The Medicines Commission accepted Upjohn's arguments and recommended that Halcion could continue to be used, provided treatment was limited to a dose of one eighth of a milligram (four to eight times less than those used in Holland) for a maximum period of ten days. In spite of this advice from the Government's most senior advisory body, the MCA refused to accept the Commission's recommendation.

The extraordinary saga continued. Upjohn then exercised its right to another form of appeal. It is called the "Person Appointed Panel" in which an expert, or in this case a group of independent experts, reconsider the evidence. They came to exactly the same conclusion as the Medicines

Commission. Yet again the MCA refused to accept it!

At one of his regular staff meetings I attended many years earlier, Sir Henry Yellowlees, the Chief Medical Officer, described his Department of Health and Social Security as the "Department of Stealth and Total Obscurity." Whether this was a Yellowlees original I do not know, but it very well described the MCA's handling of the Halcion affair. There had been several independent appraisals of the safety of Halcion since the van der Kroef incident in 1979. The CSM had agreed the reactions were dose-related and that this accounted for their rarity in the UK where the recommended dose was quite small. Several government bodies in other countries, including Holland, had come to the same conclusion. The Company had convened a group of independent experts from a wide range of disciplines, including a number of distinguished psychiatrists, who had also agreed. The Medicines Commission had called for a reassessment of their own material by an experienced assessor from the staff of the MCA itself and this had contradicted the conclusions in the MCA's original assessment. The Commission had recommended that Halcion could be reinstated with certain restrictions. Finally, the "Person Appointed Panel" had confirmed that this was the correct decision.

It is inconceivable that some medically qualified officials of the MCA could seriously believe they were right and everybody else wrong. It seems more likely that the decision to ban the drug had already been made long before the hearing. If this was true, why subject all the people involved to hundreds of hours of unnecessary work? The MCA officials could easily have given the true reasons behind the decision and nobody would have held it against them. The most logical explanation is that the civil servants advising the Minister had already decided that an example should be made of Halcion as a non-essential drug (which it probably was), the removal of which would set a precedent for further cuts in the list of drugs supplied by the NHS. The Upjohn Company lost millions of dollars and the MCA its credibility.

On September 25th 1997, the Chief Medical Officer of the Department of Health appeared on television apparently endorsing a recommendation that people should eat less meat if they want to reduce their risk of cancer. No evidence had been published or was presented to the public in the broadcast and neither he nor an equivalent official from the Department of Agriculture was prepared to defend the decision when invited to do so in *Newsnight* on the same evening. We were advised to limit our daily intake of meat to three ounces and to eat vegetable dishes "garnished" with meat! Looking back at my experiences with the pill, anaesthetic jaundice, whooping cough vaccine and Halcion, and witnessing as an outsider the shambles of the CSM's latest gaffe over the pill and the confusion about BSE, I can only shake my head in disbelief. Although I would not feed beef burgers to my grandchildren, I shall enjoy my weekly treat of mushrooms and chips "garnished" with a ten-ounce rump steak.

This is an appropriate moment to recall again, the meeting at the National Academy of Science in Washington in 1970 (Chapter 7) where it was concluded that the scientific advisers and staff of a national centre must be *"free to seek the truth wherever that may lie"* and that *"direct involvement in regulatory decisions may be contradictory to the scientific role of the Centre's staff and such involvement must be absolutely avoided."*

As a government employee I had to defend findings from studies that I had personally conducted and which were potentially of considerable scientific and public interest, against arrogant administrators who drew conclusions that better fitted their ideas about what to tell the Minister. In this book I have described three of these situations - the pill and thrombosis, halothane anaesthesia and jaundice and brain damage caused by the whooping cough vaccine. On each occasion the credibility of the Department and its advisory committees was severely damaged. More recently we have seen a re-play of the oral contraceptive blunder and have listened to seemingly authoritative claims and counter-claims about the alleged risks of BSE and genetically engineered foods. Scientists and policy makers each have their jobs to do, but their jobs must be separated. Scientific advice may be impeccable but impossible to implement on economic grounds. The views of both groups may be perfectly correct but scientists should not be involved in deciding what the policy should be and the policy makers must not be allowed to tamper with the science.

11 Please don't tell the patient!

After the practolol disaster, the CSM endorsed the need for improved methods of post-marketing surveillance (PMS) but without stipulating who should do it. This omission, exploited by the pharmaceutical industry, opened the floodgates to pseudo-scientific promotional exercises and abuse of patients' trust in their GPs. For ten years I campaigned intensively against so-called "PMS" by doctors who accept bribes from drug companies to prescribe new drugs (at taxpayers' expense) and subject their patients to avoidable risk under the pretence they are contributing to safer medicines. A doctor must not change a patient's treatment deliberately so he can participate in a marketing exercise. In any medical experiment the patient must give fully informed consent – in writing – and must be warned about the possible risks. There is always a small chance it will prove to be more dangerous than its predecessors, but this can only be confirmed by prolonged monitoring by an independent agency having no financial stake. GPs should be aware they may be sued if a patient is harmed by a drug and has not been told that she was in a PMS study.

There are three ways in which a drug company can promote a new product. The first, and in my view the only acceptable one, is that it is a novel and worthwhile treatment and has the backing of publications in widely circulated medical journals. In these circumstances the drug may almost sell itself. It establishes its role on scientific evidence alone without the need for free gifts or other inducements to prescribe it.

The second method is to set up a "Phase IV clinical trial." To understand this, it is necessary to explain briefly the four phases in the clinical development of a new drug. After satisfying themselves on the results of animal testing that a new chemical substance is likely to be safe in man, Phase I experiments are often conducted by the drug's inventors on themselves or on carefully monitored healthy volunteers such as medical students. This is potentially risky and can only be done if medical help and sophisticated equipment for resuscitation are on standby; at least one volunteer has died during an early experiment with a new drug. Phase I studies test the way the drug is handled in the body, how it is metabolised and excreted and what doses are tolerated. If nothing untoward occurs, it is then put into Phase II studies in which the investigators test the responses of "real" patients suffering from the disease the drug aims to treat. They must be fully informed volunteers who are completely free to refuse to enter the trial if they so wish. If the drug seems to have some degree of efficacy and is well tolerated, it will then pass to Phase III trials. These are full-scale clinical trials which may involve several hundred patients. Their responses are usually compared with those of patients treated with other drugs or with 'placebo' tablets that do not contain any active drug. I referred in the last chapter to my belief that the choice of comparative treatment should not be left to the manufacturer and should normally be the best alternative treatment currently available rather than a placebo. These three stages are co-ordinated by medically qualified company employees and conducted by independent clinicians. In the UK the results of all three phases are submitted to the Medicines Control Agency and scrutinised by the Committee on Safety of Medicines. If satisfactory, a licence is granted and the drug is marketed. This is the point of greatest risk. If the company has been economical with the truth or the Licensing Authority has failed to spend enough time challenging the data presented to it, thousands of patients may be treated without close supervision. Some of them could suffer severely before a new hazard is recognized. However, the present screening arrangements do provide a fair measure of safety and accidents are rare.

A Phase IV trial is started only after a drug has been licensed for sale. It often amounts to little more than a sampling exercise to introduce doctors to a new product. Some phase IV trials may test novel applications of an established product such as a modified dose regimen or the treatment of a disorder not previously regarded as an "indication" for the drug. They are usually of short duration. The company provides the doctor with free supplies of the drug and a protocol for the study. It encourages him to "recruit" patients who will be treated for a limited period while the doctor monitors the results and reports them back to the company in return for a fee. The company hopes that, having become "product-aware," the doctor will then continue to prescribe the drug for the same patients and for others who were not in the original trial. In this way the cost of the trial is rapidly recouped. Phase IV trials are often managed by company representatives. Once the doctor has agreed to participate in the study, the "rep" is guaranteed access to the doctor's office while reps from other companies may be turned away.

In one of our early PEM studies we arranged with the manufacturer, who was conducting a Phase IV study, to let us have a list of the names and addresses of all the doctors taking part in their study. We wanted to exclude these doctors from the PEM study to avoid overloading them. The company's list included about half of all the doctors whom we identified as prescribers of the drug in the whole country during the first few months after its release for sale, illustrating how effective this method of promotion can be.

A variation on this theme is for the company to set up, sometimes through a contract organisation, a so-called "PMS" study in which the GP prescribes the drug on normal NHS prescription forms and then sends follow-up reports to the company, receiving a fee for registering each patient in the study and for each follow-up report. The fee may be £15 or even more for each of several reports on each patient, and additional fees for supplementary reports. Inducements of various kinds may be offered other than cash. They have included invitations to "symposia" (e.g. golfing weekends in Scotland), air-miles (or trips to the Riviera) and electronic organisers. The study protocols may be open-ended so the patient sometimes takes the drug longer than may be necessary while the doctor continues to draw fees for follow-up reports. There are no "controls" with which to compare the new treatment and there is often a risk that patients who do not need the drug at all may be entered into the study. It may involve a change of treatment from a drug with a long and satisfactory safety record to one which turns out to have unexpected and life-threatening side effects. The cost to the taxpayer of the drug prescribed more than covers the money paid to the doctor. The final irony is that, while the doctor is being paid handsomely by the drug company, the patient, unless in an exempt category, pays the prescription charge! Patients in such trials should be aware that all post-marketing studies conducted by drug companies are promotional and they all carry some risk. Patients are not usually told that the change of treatment has been made so they can be entered into a company PMS scheme and they are certainly not volunteers. Scientifically the studies are almost uniformly valueless, as a survey by the staff of the Medicines Control Agency has demonstrated.[59] Payment or substantial gifts as an inducement to prescribe new drugs or provide information for commercial purposes should be as repugnant to doctors as it would be to their patients, if they knew what was happening to them.

In June 1987, the late Dennis Burley and I organised a seminar as part of the 6th International Meeting of Pharmaceutical Physicians in Brighton. In my talk I emphasised that promotional PMS and market research must not be confused with genuine medical research.

Promotional studies in non-volunteers had no part to play in drug safety monitoring. At another meeting of the Pharmaceutical Computer Club, also in Brighton the same year, Dr. Frank Wells counter-attacked on behalf of the Association of the British Pharmaceutical Industry (ABPI):

> "Much has appeared in the paramedical press recently referring to Prescription Event Monitoring (PEM) particularly in the light of the VAMP and AAH Meditel initiatives. As is well known, Professor Bill Inman of the Drug Safety Research Unit at Southampton wrote last month to all general practitioners arguing that the computer initiatives *which he quite wrongly ascribes to the pharmaceutical industry* (my italics) could lead to fragmentation of the procedure necessary to detect serious adverse drug reactions."

He was referring to two organisations that provided computer equipment and software enabling general practitioners to store patients' records electronically. VAMP, or Value Added Medical Products, had been set up with a great deal of encouragement from the Association of the British Pharmaceutical Industry (ABPI), and AAH Meditel was a similar organisation which had its origins in the coal industry – Allied Anthracite Holdings! Intercontinental Medical Statistics (IMS) and several other companies are also active in this field. If, for example, four organisations were competing for information about the first ten thousand patients who used a new drug, the detection of a hazard might take four times longer or it might even be missed completely because the results would not be pooled. None of the commercial organisations that pay doctors to do PMS has, to my knowledge, ever issued any warning about a major hazard detected in one of their studies.

The statement by Frank Wells was odd considering various initiatives by individual drug companies. Squibb, for example, had provided computers to three thousand GPs to conduct PMS on their product Capoten. Ciba-Geigy had supplied computers to more than two hundred practices. Bristol-Myers had loaned computers to GPs doing studies for them. ABPI's view was that the future for PMS lay in drug-company studies and I shall show why it is difficult to avoid the conclusion they successfully persuaded the authorities that this was indeed the way forward.

On the question of contracts between GPs and drug companies, Wells said:

> "We believe that data generated by a doctor on behalf of an individual pharmaceutical company in connection with a specific product must be exclusive to the company concerned. That exclusivity should not exceed a period of, say, five years from the conclusion of the project, but is an exclusivity which a pharmaceutical company has a right to expect."

This was quite unacceptable. It would prevent a doctor from passing information to independent research workers such as the DSRU, who did not have a vested interest in the particular product. (No data would ever be granted such exclusivity by the DSRU.) It would prevent participants in the company PMS study from sharing their results with colleagues or from publishing adverse experiences if they disagreed with the way the company was handling the information. Drug companies are only interested in quick results they can use to their commercial advantage. The majority of their studies are never published either because they produce no evidence that the drug is superior to its competitors or because it may have been less effective or produced more side-effects. If patients find out they have been drawn into a PMS study, they should ask their doctor precisely what use is being made of their medical records. Patients may be prepared to allow their records to be used for genuine research to help others, but few would be happy if they knew their experiences with treatment were to be locked away in company files for five years as Wells had suggested. Patients have an absolute right to insist their records should not be revealed to VAMP, AAH Meditel, the MCA, the DSRU or anyone else if that is the way they feel.

In an article in the *Guardian* in 1987 James Erlichman referred to an interview with Ian Collins, Marketing Director of VAMP Health, who said that:

> "If VAMP, when sifting its data from GPs, discovers another potential Thalidomide or Opren, it will sell the life saving information to the DHSS on a cost plus basis. Nothing in business is free," said Mr. Collins.[60]

I am not sure exactly what was meant by "cost-plus" and know how newspaper sub-editors "adjust" stories from their reporters, but I found this hard to swallow because data are collected for VAMP by responsible doctors who I am sure would want to transmit a message of such importance to the authorities immediately, and would not be pleased to know it might be sold to the authorities..

In November 1987, IMS International circulated a prospectus to clients in the drug industry. The cost of a ten thousand patient study would be £900,000, rising by 25-50% if comparisons were made with other drugs. Doctors would receive a £5 registration fee for each patient, and £5 for each follow-up report. If, for example, the protocol required five follow-up reports for each patient the doctor would earn £30 per patient. Since adverse events are rare, most reports would take only a few seconds to write. The fees mentioned in this document were modest in comparison with some more recent figures quoted in company PMS proposals.

In 1988 I published, both in a book and in the DSRU's house journal *PEM News,* hard evidence that company-sponsored Post-Marketing Surveillance (PMS) was resulting in gross over-prescribing of some new drugs.[61,62] The most striking example was a new anti-arthritis drug the CSM had provisionally recommended should be used only for the treatment of rheumatoid arthritis. It is unlikely any individual doctor would be attending more than perhaps a dozen patients with active rheumatoid arthritis at any one time. Perhaps three or four of them might be suitable for the new drug. We identified most of the first twenty thousand patients who had received prescriptions for this drug very soon after its launch. Most of the GPs had prescribed it for less than six patients. A small group of thirty-four of the country's heaviest prescribers, however, accounted for three thousand of the twenty thousand prescriptions in our sample. The average number of patients treated by each doctor in this small group was ninety and one of them had prescribed the drug for two hundred and twenty-eight patients! This could have meant that perhaps one in every ten patients in this particular doctor's practice had been prescribed a new drug that had been unnecessary for virtually all of them, and in spite of the restrictions recommended by the CSM. Since we had collected prescriptions for only a few weeks, it is more than likely these doctors have since prescribed the drug for many more patients than had appeared in our sample. The same "top prescriber" was also the country's leading prescriber of a new heart drug, accounting for a staggering total of one hundred and nine of the first three thousand four hundred patients ever to be prescribed it in the whole of England! A doctor employed by the manufacturer of the arthritis drug made no secret of the fact that GPs were being paid a three-figure fee for each patient included in the promotion. I wrote in PEM News:

"These findings are very disturbing because it is clear that some doctors have prescribed for far more patients than could possibly be monitored. If such a drug turned out unexpectedly to be as dangerous as practolol or thalidomide, there could be several "victims" in a single medical practice, possibly patients who have little need for the new drug."

What an understatement! So long as a patient's current treatment is effective and free from side-effects it is clearly bad medical practice to make any non-essential change that may expose her to unforeseen hazards. If the proposed PMS study was a genuine attempt to provide data for ensuring safety, this could only mean the drug company had accepted, quite correctly, that there may indeed be unknown risks as with all new drugs. Obviously the company cannot then claim the drug is of proven safety; if it was there would be no need to do the study! If the doctor genuinely believes the new treatment is going to have significant advantages in efficacy, and has not allowed the promise that he is to be paid to cloud his judgement, he too must accept that there is also some risk, however small he hopes it may be. This is why, if there is to be any deliberate change of treatment as a result of an approach by a drug company, the purpose of the study must be explained to the patient and the patient must sign a form of consent showing that the nature of the study and possible risks and benefits have been explained to her. The doctor should countersign the consent form and give a copy to the patient, and should ensure that the patient is comprehensively indemnified by the drug company against any possible injury. Doctors who have participated in studies without obtaining informed consent should check that their malpractice insurance will cover them if something has gone wrong and particularly if any long-delayed effects such as cancer subsequently emerge.

The medical directors of many companies have admitted to me they do not regard sponsored studies as an effective means of obtaining information about safety. I have met most of them over the years and have yet to find one who could look me in the eye and say that such activities are not promotional. Many of them prefer PMS to be conducted independently by bodies such as the DSRU. I wrote:

> "There are only two national, non-commercial schemes. Both record events which occur during normal day-to-day medical practice. Neither involve changing a patient's treatment deliberately. To do so in order to take part in a promotional study for which there is financial reward raises important scientific, ethical and legal questions which do not seem to have been adequately and publicly debated."

There was a brisk press response to this publication. Dr. Jane Richards, head of the British Medical Association's Prescribing Committee, was reported to have demanded that their joint protocols with the ABPI should be looked at again because, as she said with typical Jane Richards candour, "There is scope for abuse like merry hell." The Medical Defence Union said that GPs should make sure there was a responsible body of medical opinion in support of a new drug before changing a patient's treatment or "they could find themselves in very hot water." At a press interview I proposed that all current post-marketing studies designed to promote sales should stop immediately until the doctor's and patient's legal position and the ethical issues had been sorted out. I went on to propose that drug companies must publish a list of all commercial studies they had completed and that the results of all the studies, good or bad, must be published. Doctors must obtain fully informed consent and should not include individual patients in more than one study at a time. They should limit the number of volunteers enrolled in a trial to five or six so they can all be properly monitored Doctors must be convinced by publications in reputable journals and not by what the representatives tell them.

I became a doctor in the belief I was joining an honourable profession where the first and last consideration was the welfare of patients and not whether I could make money out of them. I believe this is so for the great majority of colleagues. As we shall see later, however, most of my attempts to persuade the industry and the authorities to stop this practice were a failure. Patients who suffer a serious adverse reaction and discover they have been put into a trial without being a fully informed volunteer should consider litigation. Unfortunately many of them will be old and will not be able to afford to do so. Until the law is changed the doctors are doing nothing that is strictly illegal; they are merely unworthy of their patients' trust.

About this time the Ministry of Health had invited bids for the old Children's Hospital at Bursledon, near Southampton. It was being used as a weekly boarding hospital and school for children with special needs, but had at one time housed some of the children who were most seriously disabled by thalidomide. It suited the needs of the DSRU admirably but at least £1 million would be required for a bid to succeed. I had hoped that the six British-based drug companies could be counted on for substantial help, but the ABPI advised companies not to co-operate in view of my recent revelations about promotional studies which they claimed was damaging the drug industry. The heads of the six company medical departments expressed dismay at this response, but told me there was nothing they could do since the sales departments controlled the budgets. Bill Cox and I therefore set off for the United States to see if we could raise the funds. We soon discovered we had been preceded by a letter from ABPI which had been circulated to all companies.

"We understand that Professor WHW Inman, Director of the Drug Safety Research Unit (DSRU) at Southampton, UK, is currently visiting the United States of America, and whilst there is visiting a number of pharmaceutical companies. We wish to draw to your attention the text of part of the current edition of PEM News which is published by the DSRU, and which is circulated to all prescribing doctors in the United Kingdom. The text, which is attached, has been widely reported to the press here to the damage of both UK and US companies, many of whom are conducting effective post-marketing surveillance studies."

This letter from ABPI caused considerable offence among doctors working for US companies and almost certainly helped rather than hindered our fund-raising effort. We raised more than £1 million fairly easily in the US and within weeks our bid for the Children's Hospital was successful.

My attack on promotional PMS was taken up in a widely publicised programme on Channel 4's *Checkout* in August 1991. ABPI and the MCA declined invitations to participate, but Stephen Dorrell, then a Conservative Health Under-Secretary, did give a brief interview saying that patients could be completely confident their doctors could handle such matters. I emphasised that studies must be "non-interventional," meaning the doctor must not deliberately intervene or change a patient's treatment to enter them into a drug company study. I also repeated my view that all studies, whether conducted before or after marketing, must only be on fully-informed volunteers. Several GPs in the programme described the gifts they had been offered such as video cameras and foreign holidays, to encourage them to participate in PMS. Representatives from drug companies openly admitted these studies were promotional. Nobody was able to explain how it might be possible to reconcile "non-intervention" with the fact that thousands of patients had started treatment with new drugs only after the doctor had agreed to accept money to do trials for a drug company or a contract research organisation. Joe Collier, the Editor of *Drug and Therapeutics Bulletin*, asked how the MCA could reasonably be expected to "sponsor" the industry and protect patients at the same time.

The arguments continued in various newspapers. Dr. Frank Wells of ABPI, challenged my statement that patients should give fully informed consent. He said that

"This is incompatible with one of the basic principles behind PMS, which is that doctors taking part in a PMS study should prescribe for their patients in as near to normal prescribing conditions as possible."

He was quite right in one sense; conditions must be as near normal as possible. This is why PMS must be non-interventional and why it must not affect treatment in any way, either by influencing the selection of suitable patients or changing existing treatment. PMS, however, must be retrospective and the information collected must have been recorded in the patient's notes *before the doctor was approached by the investigator*.

Wells also challenged my advice that patients should seek evidence that the trial drug is better than any previous medication. He said:

"It may or may not be, but in the opinion of the doctor the treatment which is being prescribed is the treatment of choice for that particular patient at that particular time."

It is difficult to understand how this could be true when a doctor had started to treat fifty or more patients with a new drug within a space of a few days. How could he have had any opinion about its value when it had been marketed so recently? All he would know is what the company would have told him.

The lid was finally blown off the credibility of drug company PMS by a "Newsletter" distributed to doctors by the Integrated Network for Computer Administration (INCA). I shall quote at length from this outrageous document:

> "INCA has strong contacts with the Department of Health, with GP computer suppliers representing over 90% of computerised practices and with the leading authorities throughout all areas of healthcare computing. Nor is it without significance, points out INCA's Joint Managing Director Garth Gunston, that INCA is part of the giant pharmaceutical distribution Group AAH, a £1.5 billion Company which already has the most advanced health care on-line ordering network in Great Britain."
>
> "A recent survey suggests that a GP could earn up to £70 for half an hour's work by completing a batch of PMS forms in a single session. A single report takes an average of three minutes and the fee payable is £7. On this basis, 10 reports completed in a single session would generate fee payments of £70"

The document then continued to invite doctors to try out Glaxo's new migraine treatment, Imigran (sumatriptan). Incredibly it began:

> "Let INCA do your PMS reporting for you. If you are a sumatriptan prescriber, but have no time for submitting PMS reports, INCA's Clinical Research Assistants will visit your practice and still let you earn the £35 per patient allowed under the PMS Code!"[63]

One can conjure up a picture of INCA's "Clinical Research Assistant" (who might have donned a white coat for maximum effect) rifling through the patient's confidential records. The newsletter described an interview with a doctor who said he had no difficulty recruiting migraine patients. I wondered how his patients would have reacted if they had seen the newsletter first?

By 1991 I was so concerned about the way patients' trust in doctors and drug companies was being abused in pseudo-scientific PMS studies, that I decided we should undertake a massive survey of prescribing, based on the hundreds of thousands of prescriptions we had collected during the DSRU's studies. Its purpose was to estimate the extent to which over-prescribing by a minority of doctors might be distorting the overall pattern of prescribing of new drugs and how much it might account for the fact that at least thirty per cent of doctors to whom we sent Prescription-Event Monitoring (PEM) questionnaires did not return them. We needed to learn more about the prescribers themselves, particularly when and where they had qualified as a doctor. One theory was that medical schools overseas might not teach the importance of cautious prescribing of new drugs. It also seemed possible that older doctors might be more cautious in their acceptance of new drugs or participation in promotional studies than younger ones.

We included twenty-seven drugs we had studied between 1984 and 1991 and prescriptions written for more than half a million patients by twenty-eight thousand GPs. During this seven-year period, nearly three thousand million prescriptions would have been written in England and Wales for drugs of all kinds, so our large sample nevertheless represented only a small fraction of all prescriptions. There is no reason to believe the GPs we identified as heavy prescribers changed their habits significantly during this period, and the data that follows represents only a fraction of their total prescribing. One prescription commonly included only one month's treatment and could have been repeated several times. We can only guess how much some of them were paid for participation in promotional studies during this seven-year period or subsequently. The results of our survey were startling and the publication in the *Lancet* with my computer manager, Gill Pearce, is the one that I believe to be the most important in my thirty years in drug safety work.[64]

We divided the doctors into six groups according to the number of prescriptions for one or more of the new drugs appearing in our samples. Group 1 had prescribed none of the drugs; Group 2 had prescribed at least one of them for up to fifteen patients, and so on in multiples of fifteen patients up to Group 6 who had prescribed for sixty or more patients. The reason for choosing fifteen-patient intervals was that this was the largest number of patients doctors were supposed to include in any one commercial study. We had not been surprised to find that some GPs had prescribed for exactly fifteen, thirty, forty-five or sixty patients, suggesting they had more than one "study" going at a time or possibly that some of them were prescribing for their partners' patients or using their partners' prescription pads.

Through our "window" in their prescribing we confirmed that excessively heavy prescribing was limited to comparatively few GPs. Twenty-two per cent of the doctors in Group I who had prescribed none of these twenty-seven new drugs were obviously cautious prescribers or were satisfied with the range of drugs already available. The top two prescribing groups in our sample, who had prescribed a new drug to more than forty-five or more than sixty patients respectively (Groups 5 and 6), comprised only two hundred and fifty-one doctors out of about twenty-eight thousand GPs in the whole sample. The drug companies would no doubt regard them as "super-prescribers." Collectively they had accounted for thirty-eight thousand treatments! Our study of each drug had covered a very short period, often only a few weeks, so their total contribution to the nation's drug costs could be relatively large. Our sample of half a million prescriptions represented only about one in every six thousand prescriptions for drugs of all kinds, new and old, written in England while our studies were in progress. How long some doctors continued with the company PMS studies and were paid to "recruit" new patients after we had finished collecting our samples is not known.

I had expected the younger GPs might be more likely to use new drugs than their older colleagues, but I was quite wrong. At the two extremes, those in Group 1 who had prescribed none of the new drugs had qualified on average about 1980 (four to seven years before our samples were collected); the moderate prescribers in Group 2 had qualified on average about 1972 (twelve to nineteen years earlier) and those in the top four heavy prescribing groups (groups 3 to 6) had, on average, qualified about 1968 (sixteen to twenty three years earlier). This result could not have been biased by only a very small percentage by the inclusion of some young doctors who had only recently become GPs. It seemed possible that modern teaching in medical schools might have made doctors more aware of the potential dangers of new drugs or more sceptical of the stories told to them by drug company representatives. Very few female doctors appeared in the samples, especially the heavy prescribing ones. This could easily be accounted for by the high proportion of female GPs working only part-time.

The other main finding was the relation between heavy prescribing of new drugs and the country in which the doctor obtained his or her first qualification. Group 1, the group that had not prescribed any of the drugs, included only thirteen per cent of overseas doctors, contrasting with over forty per cent in Groups 3 to 6. Dr. Paramjit Gill and colleagues, working on data from twenty five thousand individuals in ten thousand households provided by the General Household Survey for 1983 to 1991, almost the same period as that covered by our study, have shown that about one third more patients of Indian or Pakistani origins receive prescriptions when they consult their doctors than do non immigrant patients.[65] This result fits very well with ours.

We wondered whether the large proportion of overseas doctors, mostly from the Asian sub-continent, in the heavy prescribing groups, could reflect differences in teaching or less experience in handling the sales tricks employed to sell expensive western medicines. There was no way that forty-two per cent of the need for these new drugs could be concentrated in ten per cent of the practices; diseases do not vary to such an extent. We concluded:

> "Irrespective of the underlying reasons for the very large variations we have found in the use of recently marketed drugs (and variations in medical need cannot be one of them), there is no justification for expensive promotional studies that expose patients to the unforeseen hazards of new drugs in numbers that are far too large to be adequately monitored by individual doctors."

Several months earlier, before the publication of the results of our prescribing survey, the Minister of Health, Dr. Brian Mawhinney, had visited the DSRU and had shown considerable interest in my presentation of the results of our survey, yet unpublished. David Finney, one of our Trustees, also got in touch with Jack Ashley, and I followed this up with background information and help with the draft of his speech for a House of Lords debate on the Pharmaceutical Industry on April 28th, 1993.[66]

This debate was opened by Lord Hunter of Newington whom I had known thirty years earlier as Chairman of Derrick Dunlop's clinical trials sub-committee. Lord Hacking produced some startling statistics for the cost of the health service that had risen from about £2,000 million in 1970 to £36,000 million in 1992 and was predicted to reach £55,000 million by the year 2000. He did not, however, reveal to their Lordships the cost of the drugs that are prescribed (more than £4,000 million per year on GP prescriptions in England). Lord Rea, the House of Lords' only GP, made a strong plea that GPs should learn to use perhaps half a dozen drugs in each category, rather than to "jump into prescribing the latest preparation as soon as it comes on the market." Lord Ashley acknowledged the nice things that several noble lords had said about the drug industry but then said:

"I intend to highlight grave misgivings in regard to the surveillance of drugs to ensure safety. Some of the doctors are in danger of jeopardising the health of patients and even imperilling their lives. That is a scandalous situation which calls for urgent action by the government, the medical profession and the pharmaceutical industry. I am indebted for much of my information to Professor Bill Inman, who was the pioneer of the yellow card reporting system on adverse reactions and the originator of prescription event monitoring which is supported by four-fifths of Britain's GPs, many of whom do a great deal of work without payment.

Some companies are carrying out their own drug surveillance, an idea put forward some eight years ago by a working party, and which at first sight seems very reasonable. What is wrong with people carrying out their own drugs surveillance? What is unreasonable is the hidden objective of some companies. The first urgent danger signals should be flying when we learn that patients do not have to be fully informed volunteers giving their written consent. Why should some doctors participate in such potential malpractice? It is because they are offered inducements to take part in these commercial trials."

Jack Ashley then went on to quote from the INCA letter I have already referred to, describing it as a "blatant encouragement to doctors to supplement their incomes in this way." He quoted extensively from the results of our prescription survey and from the papers I had published on inappropriate prescribing:

> "These company trials mock scientific practice. The trials are an outrage which should be stopped by the Government and by the medical profession. Patients' informed consent must be made compulsory and the number of patients any one doctor can include in a trial should be limited."

Baroness Cumberledge, Parliamentary Under-Secretary of the Department of Health, responded:

> "Lord Ashley can rest assured that every new drug is as safe as we can make it. Those drugs undergo the most scrupulous scrutiny. Existing products on the market are carefully monitored."
>
> "Clearly every drug has the potential to do harm and clinical trials must run a minute element of risk. I do not recognise the picture painted by the noble Lord, Lord Ashley of Stoke. The Noble Lord has asked for a very full reply this afternoon. I am unable to give that but am willing to discuss with the noble Lord, on another occasion, the views that he has."

Lord Ashley then asked her if she had taken the trouble to read the material the DSRU had sent to Dr. Mawhinney. She had not. Later she wrote to him apologising that she had confused the yellow card system with company PMS and offering to meet both of us. This confusion illustrated the point I have made several times about the poor quality of briefing of ministers. She could not have been wider off the mark.

The meeting was delayed for some months because Jack Ashley went into hospital to have a cochlear implant in the hope of restoring some hearing. When we next met later in 1993, he was already beginning to hear some of the discussion, although still using a portable visual display system and a transcriber who operates it from a distance during debates in the House.

In the meantime on June 7th, the Conservative Secretary of State, Dr. Brian Mawhinney, wrote:

Richmond House
June 7th 1993 Dear Prof. Inman,

Thank you for your letter of 19th April and for providing me with further information about your studies. I am sorry you have not had an earlier reply.

The Government is concerned by your data which have shown that, over the past few years, some doctors have prescribed new medicines for large numbers of patients in post-marketing surveillance (PMS) studies, and agrees that this is undesirable.

Initiatives in three areas are, we believe, capable of addressing the problems. Firstly the introduction to prescribing, analysis and cost (PACT) data, and appointment of family health services authorities' (FHSA's) prescribing advisers, has meant that significant over-prescribing is now being identified and action taken against persistent offenders. PACT data are currently being improved with a view to highlighting use of new drugs. Secondly, proposals for revising and strengthening the existing post-marketing surveillance guide-lines are under discussion. One of the proposed changes is to place a limit on the number of patients that may be entered into a study by a single doctor. Other changes are designed to improve the sci-entific value of PMS studies and minimise promotional aspects. Finally the EC Advertising Directive is presently being implemented into UK law and will provide controls on inducements to prescribe. Thus there will soon be a statutory basis on which action will be taken against those who offer to accept inducements to prescribe. We shall be monitoring the effects of these measures on the problems you describe.

Thank you again for drawing these issues to my attention.

I hope this is helpful, Yours sincerely
Brian Mawhinney.

At first sight it seemed I might have made some small progress after many years of struggle, but Dr. Mawhinney had dodged the two most important issues. He did not comment on whether patients should be fully informed volunteers nor on the justification for changing existing effective treatment that was of proven safety and efficacy. He left the door open for doctors who are prepared to prescribe a new (and often much more expensive) drug for patients who may not need it, who are not given any choice, and who are not aware the doctor is being paid to do so by a drug company.

In September 1993, our paper was published in the *Lancet*. We successfully avoided publicity that might have led to criticism on "ethnic" grounds. Several Asian doctors congratulated us for having had the courage to draw attention to a problem they were very well aware of and attributed to a minority of their compatriots. There were even signs that some influential people were beginning to come out in support. Sir William Asscher, who had now retired as Chairman of the CSM, told the

Independent that drug company studies were often just a "marketing exercise." He criticised them for being informal, in the sense that there were no rigid protocols and the companies were not required to publish their findings; but he did not go nearly far enough.

It seemed possible that the Government's reluctance to take action against this practice stemmed from anxiety that they might antagonise the ethnic minorities within the medical profession. The close links between overseas doctors and company sales representatives was illustrated by a rather curious letter I received from Paddy Ashdown, Leader of the Liberal Democrats, that had obviously been sent to me in error in the mistaken belief I was an Asian GP. He invited me to dinner at the House of Commons! He expressed concern about the uncaring attitude adopted by the Prime Minister (John Major) and the medical manpower implications of the European Community which might place Asian doctors at a disadvantage. The letter said that only a limited number of people were to be invited and a slip was attached which would be honoured on a first-come-first-served basis. The price of a ticket was £95. This slip of paper carried a rather startling message:

> "The function is not limited to Asians and you may invite non-Asians including Pharmaceutical Company representatives."

If places at table were so limited, why single out drug reps as people that the Asian doctors might wish to bring with them? Was it possible the doctor might see this as an opportunity to return past hospitality from the drug rep? Was it possible drug reps were the only friends the Asian doctors were supposed to have? Perhaps Paddy Ashdown felt that the doctor would not attend the dinner unless he could find a drug rep to pay the £95. I am sure Paddy Ashdown must have been advised about what I had learned when I worked for ICI forty years earlier. Doctors from the Asian sub-continent were specifically targeted by drug reps.

One senior Asian doctor, a postgraduate tutor in general practice, phoned the DSRU and then wrote at length, setting out the reasons why he disagreed with one of my theories. I had suggested there might be different standards of training in various countries. He has encouraged me to quote him at length and to reveal his name if I wished. He said it was:

> "...the specific targetting by pharmaceutical companies which causes this high level of prescribing by a small minority. I know because I have been targetted, but because of my basic beliefs I have not succumbed to the pressure. You may well ask why Asian doctors are susceptible to such pressures while the English doctors are not. In any society an individual accepts the mores of that society because he is part of that society and does not want to be alienated from it. An immigrant, whatever his attempts at integration, remains an outsider for reasons I need not go into. This is especially true if the immigrant is perceived to be a second class citizen. If an immigrant is not integrated in a society then he does not feel bound to accept the mores of that society. He will break the accepted code of the society till he is in the grey area of behaviour which may be unethical but still legal. As we well know, those in high finance, the Maxwells of this world, do this every day. I am interested in this subject not only to reduce wastage in the NHS and provide better service to the patients, but also to maintain the reputation of a large majority of Asiatic GPs who try to give a good service but get tarred with the same brush."

About the same time as the *Lancet* paper appeared, the draft guidelines for company-sponsored *Safety Assessment Of Marketed Medicines* (SAMM) were distributed by the Association of the British Pharmaceutical Industry (ABPI).[67] Some features were an improvement on previous guidelines, but not the most important ones, and they were clearly designed to encourage drug company promotional studies. The guidelines had been formulated by a working party which included representatives of the Department of Health, the British Medical Association, the Royal College of General Practitioners, and the Committee on Safety of Medicine. The ABPI is nothing more than a trade association and it should be no part of their remit to become involved in instructing doctors in ethical matters. If the *"Guidelines"* were to have any credibility, they should have been distributed by the CSM or the Department of Health rather than the pharmaceutical industry. In fairness to ABPI, their Data Sheet Compendium is probably the most reliable source of information about drugs and it is approved by the MCA. However, to include the CSM and the Department in a communication from ABPI created the impression that ABPI had official status in matters of medical ethics.

One recommendation in the SAMM guidelines was regarded by some of my supporters as a triumph for my campaign though I would lay no claim to it. Clause 3.(d) read:

"Patients must not be prescribed particular medicines in order to include them in observational cohort studies since this is unethical (see section 15 of the 'guidelines on the Practices of Ethics Committees in Medical Research involving Human Subjects,' Royal College of Physicians, 1990)."

At last they had agreed that patients' treatments must not be changed to enter them into a study and their use of the word "unethical" was a step forward. Clause 3(d) now stated very clearly that the practice I had persistently complained about for more than ten years is unethical. It remains to be seen how successful the industry will be in finding ways round this clause.

Another Clause, 3(f), stated that no patient should be entered in more than one study simultaneously. We had occasionally found patients who had been in up to four studies at the same time or in rapid succession. Any observations made in such studies would be impossible to interpret. No limit was suggested to the number of patients that might be included in a study. Clause 5(e) states:

> "A final report on the study should be sent to the MCA within three months of follow-up being completed."

No limit to the duration of any single study was stipulated. All the company needs to do is to prolong the follow-up by stretching the numbers of patients entered into the study, keeping a trickle of patients going until it is no longer profitable. Finally, clause 7(b):

> "No inducement for a doctor to participate in a SAMM study should be requested, offered or given."

I have seen a letter from a company doing a so-called "SAMM" study of a treatment for angina. It looks little different from the "PMS" studies of old. The doctor was expected to treat four patients with the new drug plus two controls with conventional nitrite treatment. For this he would receive a fee of £275 with an extra £15 thrown in if a serious adverse reaction had to be reported. It goes on to say that "Each GP could however have booklets to fill in for a maximum of 18 patients, but the ratio (new drug to old) will be maintained." Sales of the drug will cover the cost many times over. Only one thing seems probable – the results of the study, if they are ever published, will probably have little or no scientific value.

One can only be amazed that the MCA and CSM agreed that the SAMM guidelines were a sufficient safeguard, when there is no absolute limit to the number of patients for whom one doctor may prescribe one or more new drugs. There is no mention of what the patient should be told about possible side-effects. There is no guidance about patient-indemnity or compensation. Worst of all there is no instruction that would ensure that the patient must be an informed volunteer. The SAMM guidelines are partial to drug companies and lamentably inadequate; guidelines are only guidelines and not laws.

Predictably, the SAMM logo is now being used to advertise promotional studies. In September 1997, a contract house called IBRD-Rostrum mailed a "PMS news flash." It reads:

"In our most recent SAMMs study, IBRD-ROSTRUM GLOBAL, in a record time of 6 months, successfully completed enrolment of 7,500 patients nine months ahead of schedule "

The drug was a typical "me too" product competing, alongside another "me too", with the highly effective and perfectly satisfactory product, Losec, used for the treatment of digestive disorders, which has the considerable advantage of having had a successful non-commercial PEM study by the DSRU. I do not know if there is any evidence that they have any advantages in efficacy, but the competition for the first ten thousand patients which seems to have gone to IBRD-Rostrum, would be certain to delay any study by the DSRU. Patients and doctors should await Rostrum's report on their "SAMM" study with considerable interest (if such a report ever appears in a medical journal that submits offerings to referees).

The meeting with Baroness Cumberledge, arranged by Jack Ashley, took place at the end of October 1993. We were joined by John Ferguson, the new Medical Director of the Prescription Pricing Authority. The

Baroness was a good listener and seemed to share my outrage at certain aspects of the case, especially the INCA document. After the meeting, Jack Ashley wrote to say he felt that the meeting had been very useful and that she would respond positively. Her final reply, however, was depressingly negative. She said the Department was satisfied with the guidelines and its view was that consent from the patient was not required. She then, to our utter amazement, said:

> "I understand that patients' consent is not obtained for studies conducted by Professor Inman's Unit."

This was clearly what she had been told by the MCA's officials and I would not hold it against her personally. Any vestige of credibility was now swept away. This statement was deliberately misleading and it could come to haunt the officials when they are called to account in the law suits that must surely arise if patients in some future drug company study suffer severe reactions. They knew perfectly well there is no resemblance whatsoever between PEM studies set up by the DSRU and promotional studies run by drug companies. PEM is retrospective and non-interventional. Green forms are sent to the GP six or more months *after* he had first prescribed the new drug. In no way is he "recruited" into the study or encouraged by the DSRU to prescribe a particular drug. Company studies on the other hand are prospective and involve a deliberate change of treatment after the company or contract agency has asked the doctor to "recruit" patients for the study. In PEM doctors receive no payment for completing the forms, in drug company studies they only complete them if paid in cash or kind to do so. The Department's response was shameful, no words are strong enough to describe it, or the behaviour of the officials who were responsible for it.

The Department officials and the Committee know perfectly well that if patient-consent was legally required for PMS studies, they would cease to be used for drug promotion. They have the power to put a stop to these practices at a stroke of a pen. The enormous waste of resources on developing, testing and licensing "me too" products would be avoided if the manufacturers found them more difficult to sell. I touched on the way this might be achieved by modifying the patent laws earlier and how the annual saving on the annual NHS drug bill might top £2,000 million.

The ABPI and the Department tried to rubbish our survey published in the *Lancet*. They claimed we had not provided evidence that the huge volume of prescribing in some practices was the direct result of company promotional PMS studies. They were well aware that prescriptions are sent to the DSRU by the PPA on the strict understanding that the identities of doctor and patient will never be revealed. We did not cite individual companies because so many of them were involved and we had not been able to study all the drugs included in promotional studies. Obviously we could not implicate doctors who had participated in company studies because this would breach the confidence on which the whole operation of PEM depended. The Department and ABPI have records of which drugs had been included in promotional studies because the companies are bound to inform them. Legal representatives of any patient who suffers a severe adverse reaction should have little difficulty finding out if their clients have been included in promotional PMS without seeking permission. It is no part of the DSRU's duty to act as policeman.

The notion that the substantial sums paid to doctors are intended to cover their "expenses" is facile hypocrisy. New drugs should only be marketed when they have been shown, in scientific studies, to have a worthwhile margin of superiority in efficacy or safety or both. The pharmaceutical lobby carefully ensured that comparative efficacy was excluded in the drafting of the Medicines Act of 1968. Clinical trials are only large enough to reveal common side effects. Safety can only be confirmed by independent post-marketing surveillance on a large scale and not by the promoter.

The drug industry and their trade association, the ABPI, have persistently refused to accept the most important ethical principle that patients should be volunteers. That nothing is done about it reflects an unhealthy relationship between the MCA and the drug industry. The MCA is not only run as a business, it calls itself a business and, horror of horrors, the yellow card system is now officially referred to as the "Adverse Reactions Business"! Many members of the government committees who advise the MCA are consultants to the industry. They are chosen by civil servants and not, as they should be, elected by the Royal Colleges. Robust and independent characters tend not to be re-elected when their term of office finishes. The dual role of the MCA to promote the drug industry and assure safety is dangerous and unworkable.

Commercial PMS studies are most likely to be conducted on drugs which are not novel and are merely competing for a share of a lucrative market; PMS is rarely used for major "break-through" drugs. Patients receiving on-going treatment should be particularly suspicious of any sudden and unexplained change, especially with drugs for chronic diseases that are likely to be needed for months or even years, such as arthritis, stomach disorder or asthma. In the unlikely situation in which a doctor has suggested that the patient might volunteer to take part in a study, she should be told the name of the manufacturer and who will indemnify her in the event of an adverse reaction to the new drug. If patients agree to start the new treatment they should ensure that the GP will immediately report any side effects.

Early in 1964, before joining Derrick Dunlop's Committee to develop the yellow card system, I discussed with him the difficulty I thought civil servants would experience if they attempted to be loyal to a scientific group on the one hand, and the Minister of the day on the other. We had both felt it would be unlikely to work for long. I promised to "give it a whirl" (my exact words), and the whirl lasted sixteen years. After leaving the Committee, my next fourteen years of independence were dogged by antagonism and jealousy from those who were not independent, but I take some pride in the fact I had successively developed the only two non-commercial monitoring schemes operating on a country-wide basis, and left both of them "up and running" when I retired after thirty years' of drug safety work.

I have failed to persuade the medical profession to cease their involvement in promotional studies by drug companies. To patients I would say – if you should find yourself in the position I have described and have suffered any adverse drug reaction, you should make a formal complaint to the local health authority and, if you can afford it, seek legal advice. You can obtain advice from the Law Society Help Line (0171 320 5713), Action for Victims of Medical Accidents * or the College of Health‡. This book may stimulate enough concern to ensure that the struggle to correct these anomalies is continued.

* Bank Chambers, 1 London Road, Forest Hill, SE23 3TP

‡ St.Margaret's House, 21 Old Ford Road, E2 9PL

12 Lessons Learned

In 1995 I was honoured by the prestigious international Drug Information Association (DIA) with a Distinguished Career Award. The award ceremonies were to be held in Paris and I was by then too disabled by the progressive effects of the "Post-Polio Syndrome" to attend in person. As a compromise, a seven-minute film was made of my acceptance speech and shown to the audience in Paris during the award ceremony. I had been asked to recall what I thought were the main lessons I had learned during more than thirty years in drug safety monitoring. With a little thought I came up with four:

1. The need for independence.
2. The need for transparency.
3. Consideration of relative efficacy as well as relative safety.
4. Patients in prospective studies must be fully informed volunteers.

The first essential for any drug monitoring system, as with all research, is independence. Without independence it is impossible to resist pressures which would interfere with the proper conduct of the research. Obviously, in matters affecting health, it is essential to keep the public, the medical profession and official bodies informed of all important findings. However, there is nothing more damaging to the credibility of an organisation if it falls victim to premature publicity and releases information that turns out to be wrong. There are several examples in this book.

A serious mistake was made shortly before the Medicines Act of 1968 came into effect in 1971; it perpetuated the problems with the yellow card system that stemmed from lack of independence. Under the Act a Medicines Commission was set up to advise the government and to make recommendations about how drug safety assurance should be continued. The plan was that the Medicines Commission would be advised by several committees (known under the Act as Section-IV committees), one of which was to be a reconstituted Committee on Safety of Medicines which would take over from the "Dunlop Committee." The Licensing Authority (later replaced by the Medicines Control Agency) would continue to scrutinise the data obtained in animal studies and pre-marketing clinical trials to ensure that the drug company studies had been correctly carried out and no unacceptable toxicity had been detected. These are "armchair" assessments of drug company work in which the officials and the committee have taken no active part themselves. The work of the Adverse Reactions Sub-Committee on the other hand had always been focused on what happens after a new drug had been marketed. They depended on "hands on" work by myself and my staff and they based their recommendations on the information supplied in my monthly report which always included a commentary and suggestions for possible action. We in turn depended on their guidance but on no occasion since it was set up in 1964 had the Sub-Committee identified a problem that we had not already brought to their attention. If we missed an important signal it could remain undetected almost indefinitely. If we read too much into a signal, the Committee might make an inappropriate recommendation leading to withdrawal of a drug from the market.

The best course of action had been very carefully debated with the

Sub-Committee. There were only two options. The first was to give PMS separate status and greater power as a Section IV Committee in its own right. The second was for it to remain a subcommittee of the CSM. As had been clear at the Washington conference, it was essential that post-marketing research should be done by staff who were not responsible for licensing and who were free to consult appropriate people outside the Department at any time.

The first option was clearly the best; PMS should be independent of licensing. After seven years operating the yellow card scheme, most of the medical staff and some of the administrators realised it had been a mistake to place adverse reactions monitoring within the Department. We now had an opportunity to reorganise. The arguments in favour of the first option were carefully rehearsed before the crucial first meeting of the Medicines Commission. Incredibly and catastrophically, when Derrick Dunlop who had been appointed its first Chairman asked for the views of the Sub-Committee on Adverse Reactions, he was told that no change was necessary and that it need not be given the status of a separate Section IV committee! What had happened during the chairman's lunch with senior administrators before the Commission's meeting and how this catastrophic reversal arose I shall probably never find out, but any hope that we could work independently of the Licensing Authority was lost. The rug had been well and truly pulled from under my wheels!

Before this disastrous meeting of the New Commission, there had been much discussion of who should chair a newly constituted Section IV committee to work on adverse reactions. An obvious choice had been Sir Richard Doll. The administrators, however, kept this suggestion from Sir Derrick, probably because they feared Richard was likely to express independent views too forcefully for their liking. When I heard of this deliberate omission, I phoned Sir Derrick in Edinburgh a day or so before the fateful meeting. He said, "Of course we must invite Richard" and immediately did so. Richard accepted, believing as I had, that he would be chairing an independent group. My duty now lay in supporting Richard since I had unwittingly pitched him into a situation that neither of us had anticipated. My decision to stay in London delayed the introduction of the second national monitoring scheme that I was eventually able to set up in Southampton. Had it started earlier, perhaps in 1972 rather than 1980, I am sure that more of my objectives, such as establishing teaching programmes and mechanisms for epidemiological studies, might have been achieved before I retired in 1994.

The Drug Safety Research Unit DSRU has sometimes been criticised because its work has not resulted in the removal of any drug from the market. In the eyes of the press and some politicians, the banning of drugs is a benchmark of success in drug safety monitoring. Banning a drug is neither an objective nor a responsibility of an independent institution such as the DSRU. The great majority of drugs turn out to be relatively safe. Unless the adverse reactions are so bizarre they cannot fail to be recognised, all monitoring schemes will fail to detect very rare events. If, as happens quite frequently, a valuable treatment is threatened by reports of adverse reactions to it, it takes courage, experience and intellectual honesty to wait until enough convincing evidence has been collected to justify action. People conducting post-marketing research must be free to publish their findings when and only when they are ready.

Drug company medical departments must not be allowed to "filter" reports of adverse reactions. The CSM introduced a black triangle mark that had to be appended to the name of a new drug in any advertising material until they were satisfied there were no serious hazards. It should have been a red triangle to suggest possible dangers, but the industry would not agree. They could even use the black triangle promotionally as a mark of novelty.

***

My second lesson was the importance of transparency. A major criticism of the licensing and committee structure in the UK and in some other countries is that their affairs are conducted in secrecy. In the US, with its Freedom of Information Act, ordinary citizens can gain access to information held in the files of the FDA. In the UK, information supplied by drug companies is classed by the authorities as "Commercial in Confidence" because what is bad news for one company may be good news for another. From the first hours of marketing a new product, every detail of its properties, the results of clinical trials, and data on adverse reactions should be available to anybody with a need to know. The application of the Official Secrets Act to civilian medical research is ludicrous. It may be appropriate when applied to research on nerve gas or biological warfare, but it was nonsensical, for example, to try to apply it to my research on thrombosis and the contraceptive pill in the sixties.

The most serious effect of secrecy is that it allows officials to hide their mistakes and the reasons behind controversial decisions. This was illustrated by the Halcion affair. In that case a clear explanation might have salvaged the MCA's credibility; their silence shattered it. When investigating a drug safety problem, inability to assemble all the information because some of it, such as the data sent to the MCA in support of new drug applications is confidential, can be dangerous. Secrecy ruined the joint DSRU/CSM "Red Alert" scheme that might have been a considerable advance in early-warning of drug hazards.

Research results must be published and the data must always be open to inspection. Authors must make themselves available to answer criticisms. They must be able to defend their findings or to admit they might have been wrong. Official statements, especially those about a drug withdrawal, must be backed up by details about the reasons for them. Civil servants are in a position of power without personal responsibility. Frequently they become arrogant, forgetting they are servants and not masters. Their Minister may be called to account for the decision taken on their advice but few civil servants ever appear on a TV programme to defend them. I well remember discussing this problem with Bruce Royal, the first Head of the WHO monitoring scheme in Geneva. We both felt we were in danger of becoming arrogant because of the power we wielded. We had both given up direct involvement in clinical medicine, yet we were in a position where we could influence the medical practice of colleagues who had far more specialist experience than we had. We had to keep reminding ourselves that our duty lay in bringing the facts to their attention but not telling them how to practise medicine.

Some progress with feed-back of information has been made by the CSM who continue to circulate occasional leaflets in a *"Current Problems"* series that was the brain-child of one of my assistants, Paul Dendy, more than twenty years ago. This is especially important as a vehicle for feeding back information to general practitioners who are responsible for the bulk of drug prescriptions. It is informative without causing undue alarm. The corresponding publication by the DSRU was *PEM News*. This series has fallen by the wayside in recent years in favour of more "academically correct" publications in low-circulation journals. These are useful as a scientific record of the results of PEM studies but have no impact on the GPs who supply the information. GPs need information as soon as it is available and it may take many months or even several years to complete and publish a detailed report.

***

My third lesson and a message for those who shape the future of risk management, is that public health decisions must be based on complete therapeutic equations and on a clear idea of the acceptability of various levels of risk that may be taken to achieve a desired objective. The risk of treatment must never exceed the risk of the disease, so the equation must first include knowledge of the natural risks of the disease. How many people suffering from it die from it, how many with a particular symptom find it intolerable? Having determined these levels, the next stage is to determine the relative efficacy of the available treatments, including all the alternatives such as surgery, drugs, psychotherapy and so on. Finally, it is essential to know the relative safety of all the treatments available. All effective drugs have some risks. It may be possible to cure a disease with a very risky form of treatment but only to palliate it with less dangerous treatments. Heroic treatment of cancer may be acceptable to a young patient in spite of horrendous side-effects, while it might not be acceptable to an elderly person. The Medicines Act of 1968 did not require evidence of relative efficacy in the granting of product licences for sale. This omission continues to allow a significant fraction of the nation's resources to be frittered away on patenting, clinical trial, scrutiny and licensing of "me too" drugs, many of which have no advantages over earlier products and most of which are more expensive. I have tried to show how a small change to the patent laws might halve the £4,000 million GP drug bill in the United Kingdom.

***

My fourth lesson was the most important of all. I had exposed the abuse of patients' trust in doctors who put them to unnecessary risks in promotional studies organised by some drug companies, and I declared my intention to continue fighting for patients' rights to know if their doctors are changing their treatment for personal gain without first obtaining their informed consent. I reiterated my total opposition to quasi-scientific post-marketing studies, most of which are not published and none of which had uncovered a previously unrecognised side effect.

Some people thought my opposition to company studies was contrived because I wanted a monopoly for the DSRU. In reality it was because it was essential to have access to as much data as possible during the critical period when the first ten thousand or more patients are treated with a new drug. Fragmentation of records of drug treatments among more than one group of investigators will inevitably delay detection of hazards. It is essential to use the same method for all investigations so the results can be compared, one drug with another and one study with another. Studies by different companies cannot be compared because their methods are not standardised, the data is "interpreted," and the results (if any) are locked away in company or departmental files labelled "commercial, in confidence."

The short patent life of innovative new drugs produces a constant flow of "me too" drugs. They have few advantages over their competitors and the only way to promote them is by expensive mailings and visits by representatives or by "Post-Marketing Surveillance". Without these promotional exercises sales would develop too slowly to sustain the sales departments and the seven-figure salaries of their top executives. The head of one corporation was said in 1995 to have earned more than £12 million in fringe benefits such as share options.[68] This would have funded the DSRU for most of its 20-year life.

The Pharmaceutical Industry and the MCA are well aware that if patients in such studies were fully-informed volunteers, promotional PMS would stop. They are aware that if genuine new discoveries had long-term patent protection, the flow of "me too" products would diminish (saving a large fraction of GP drug costs). Competition in many industries is healthy because it encourages manufacturers to sell high quality goods at reasonable prices. Competition in the treatment of disease is a different matter. It steers doctors away from time-tested products and encourages them to take unnecessary risks. The Government, the medical profession and the public must wake up to the fact that the treatment of common conditions has become a matter of competition for markets. If the waste on "me too" drugs could be stopped, resources could be diverted to other areas of health care. The industry's argument that without "me too" drugs there would be no money to fund major advances is sheer nonsense. In this book I have shown how the authorities have failed to prevent exploitation of sick patients. It is a pity that we will have to wait until a major tragedy with a new drug undergoing promotional trials forces them to change the rules.

***

For good measure I threw in an extra lesson. It is a belief that I have always been more than willing to share with colleagues, students and staff. It is, quite simply — anything really worth doing should be fun. If it ceases to be fun, the time has come to do something about it or change jobs. I have enjoyed almost everything I have done in a long career in drug safety work, although a time came during my sixteen years in the Department of Health when the sacrifices that had to be made by me and my family and the failure to provide the Committee with the resources they needed, meant that the only sensible decision was to leave. Setting up the DSRU and developing the second national system presented a greater challenge, and was even more fun.

Very sadly I have to admit that in spite of my efforts to build bridges with people whose livelihoods depended on "business", I was slow to realise that drug companies, regulatory agencies and most seemingly independent "monitors," cannot always be depended upon to keep their noses entirely clean when their support depends on business, shareholders, balance sheets, jobs or votes. I believe I succeeded in doing this while responsible for the DSRU, largely because it was managed by a charitable trust, withheld no results, signed no contracts and relinquished no intellectual rights.

From 1948 the pharmaceutical industry prospered. Patients no longer needed to pay for their drugs and profits escalated. More recently, prescription charges increased but the flow of genuinely innovative drugs started to diminish. Many of the gaps in medical treatment were already filled and the industry was beginning to run out of steam. Most new introductions were merely "me too" variants or old patent-expired products with new brand names. Some companies formed satellites to sell their old products in pseudo-competition with the parent company. Increasingly, the industry had to rely on dubious practices to promote second-rate products. Latterly, massive mergers such as Glaxo and Wellcome, SmithKlein and Beecham and Zeneca and Astra, enabled large sections of the industry to reduce its work-force without trimming its list of products or their cost.

After Eraldin and one or two lesser catastrophes, doctors were beguiled into believing that "PMS" by drug companies was the answer to drug safety. Little of note has ever been published from drug company PMS studies. The Medicines Control Agency was set the impossible task of promoting the interests of the industry and assuring safety at the same time. It has not succeeded in curtailing promotional PMS or dealing with the ethical problems involved. Specifically, it has not insisted that patients in drug-company studies should be fully informed volunteers. Patients would be horrified if they knew they were one of hundreds of thousands whose doctors have been paid to change existing treatment or start something new.

Since 1980, the DSRU has been able to make some advances in general practice monitoring. Few really new products have emerged from pharmaceutical laboratories in recent years but we may expect to see treatments of an entirely novel kind such as gene therapy or bio-engineered products that stimulate an immune response to cancer cells. Hopefully the DSRU and other institutions will be able to develop new methods and attract new people to take over from the old timers like Herschel Jick in the USA and myself in the UK. We have done our best over many years to keep safety monitoring going on a "no strings" basis (i.e. paid for, but not controlled by industry or government). The future of drug-safety monitoring lies well away from drug companies, industrially sponsored units, government departments beholden to political parties, or consumer groups. It should be managed by scientists under the general direction of a completely independent body such as the Medical Research Council, funded by the taxpayer and not the industry. It certainly must not be controlled by bureaucrats in London or Brussels.

References

1. Inman, WHW. *Feeling Better Doctor?* (In preparation).

2. Reader, WJ. (1970). *Imperial Chemical Industries,* A History. 1870-1926. Oxford University Press.

3. Hopkinson, DAW and Watts, JC. (1963). Studies in Experimental Missile Injuries of Skeletal Muscle. Proc.Roy.Soc.Med; 56:461-8.

4. Dziemian, AJ., Mendleson, JA. and Lindsey, D. (1961). Comparison of the wounding characteristics of some commonly encountered bullets. *J.Trauma.* 1,4; 341-53.

5. McBride, WG. (1961). Thalidomide and congenital abnormalities. *Lancet* 4,1358.

6. Lenz, W. (1962). Thalidomide and congenital abnormalities. *Lancet* 1, 45.

7. Ministry of Health (1964). Deformities caused by Thalidomide. Ministry of Health Report no.112. *HMSO.* London.

8. Thromboembolic Phenomena in Women. (1962). Conference proceedings at a symposium sponsored by G.D. Searle & Co. Sept, 10th 1962.

9. Inman, WHW. (1970). Role of Drug-Reaction Monitoring in the Investigation of thrombosis and "The Pill". *British Medical Bulletin* 26.3, 248-56.

10. College of General Practitioners (1967). Oral Contraceptives and Thrombo-embolic Disease. *J.Coll.Gen.Practit.* 13, 267.

11. Medical Research Council (1967). Risk of Thromboembolic Disease in women taking oral contraceptives. *British Medical Journal.* 2. 355.

12. Inman, WHW., Vessey, MP. (1968). Investigation of deaths from pulmonary coronary and cerebral thrombosis and embolism in women of child-bearing age. *British Medical Journal.* 2, 193.

13. Vessey, MP. and Doll, R. (1968). Investigation of relation between use of oral contraceptives and thromboembolic disease. *British Medical Journal* 2,199.

14. Inman, WHW., Vessey, MP., Westerholm, B. and Engelund, A. (1970). Thromboembolic disease and the steroidal content of oral contraceptives. *British Medical Journal.* 2, 203.

15. Mann, JI., Inman, WHW. and Thorogood, M. (1976). Oral contraceptive use in older women and myocardial infarction. *British Medical Journal.* 2, 445.

16. Inman, WHW. (1979). Oral Contraceptives and fatal subarachnoid haemorrhage. *British Medical Journal*. 2. 1468.

17. Inman, WHW. (1972). The relationship between oestrogen's and progestogens and thromboembolic disease. *Menopause and Aging*. U.S. Department of Health Education and Welfare. Bethesda. Md. 71-104.

18. Greenberg, MJ. (1966). letter to *Lancet* ii.442

19. Greenberg, MJ. and Pines, A. (1967). letter to *British Medical Journal* i.563.

20. Inman, WHW., Adelstein, AM. (1969). The rise and fall of asthma mortality in England and Wales in relation to use of pressurised aerosols. *Lancet* 2.279-85.

21. Inman, WHW. (1974). Recognition of unwanted drug effects with special reference to pressurised bronchodilator aerosols. Asthma Research Council. Symposium October 1973. 191-206 FJ Parsons.

22. Stolley, PD. (1972). Asthma Mortality. Why the United States was spared an epidemic of deaths due to asthma. *American Review of Respiratory Diseases*. 105.883-90.

23. Inman, WHW. and Mushin, WW. (1974). Jaundice after Repeated Exposure to Halothane: An Analysis of Reports to the Committee on Safety of Medicines. *British Medical Journal*. 1. 5-10.

24. Walton, B et al. (1976) Unexplained hepatitis following halothane. *British Medical Journal*. 1. 171-6.

25. *Times Law Report*. Queen's Bench Division Dec 6th 1972.

26. Felix, R. and Ive, FA. (1974). Skin reactions to practolol. *British Medical Journal*. 2.333. May 11th.

27. Wright, P. (1974) Skin reactions to practolol. *British Medical Journal* 2.560. June 8th.

28. Herbst, AL., Ulfelder, H. and Poskanza, DC. (1971). *New England Journal of Medicine* 284, 878-81.

29. Smithells, RW. and Chinn, ER. (1964). Meclozine and Foetal Malformations: A Prospective Study. *British Medical Journal*. 1.217-8.

30. Smithells, RW. and Sheppard, S. (1978). *Teratology*, 17,1.31-5.

31. Edwards, J H. (1958). *British Journal of Preventive and Social Medicine* 12,

32. Gal, I., Kirman, B. and Stern, J. (1967). *Nature*, 216, 83.

33. Greenberg, G., Inman WHW., Weatherall, AC. and Adelstein, AM. (1975). British Medical Journal, *British Medical Journal*. 2. 191-2.

34. Greenberg, G., Inman, WHW., Weatherall, JAC., Adelstein, AM. and Haskey, JC. (1977). Maternal Drug Histories and Congenital Abnormalities. *British Medical Journal* 2, 853-6.

35. Joint Committee on Vaccination and Immunisation (1975). Whooping-cough Vaccine. *British Medical Journal*. 274.687.

36. National Academy of Sciences. (1971). *Report of the International Conference on Adverse Reactions Reporting Systems, October* 22-23 1970. Drug Research Board, Washington DC.

37. Finney, DJ. (1965). The Design and Logic of a Monitor of Drug Use. Journal of chronic Diseases. 18,77-98.

38. Inman, WHW. (1978). in *Epidemiological Issues in Reported Drug-Induced Illnesses - SMON and Other Examples*. Proceedings of an international symposium on 19th-21st January 1976. M. Gent and I Shigematsu (eds). 17-24.McMaster University Library Press. Hamilton, Ontario.

39. Inman, WHW. (1976). *Royal Society of Health*. 83rd Congress, Eastbourne, 29th April 1976.

40. Gross, FH. and Inman, WHW. (1977), *Drug Monitoring*. Academic Press. London.

41. Hammond, KR. (1978), Integrated facts and values in the development and regulation of drugs. in. M. Gent and I Shigematsu (eds). Epidemiological Issues in Reported Drug-Induced Illnesses - SMON and Other Examples. Proceedings of an international symposium on 19th-21st January 1976. 327-337 McMaster University Library Press. Hamilton, Ontario.

42. Collier, Joe. (1989). *The Health Conspiracy*. Century Hutchinson Ltd. London.

43. Medawar, C (1992). *Power and Dependence*. Social Audit Ltd. London.

44. Abraham, J. (1995). *Science, Politics and the Pharmaceutical Industry*. University College London (UCL) Press Ltd.

45. Inman, WHW. (ed) (1980). *Monitoring for Drug Safety*. MTP Press Ltd. Lancaster.

46. Inman, WHW. (1980). in Soda T.(ed) Drug-Induced Sufferings: Proceedings of the Kyoto Conference Against Drug-Induced Sufferings (KICADIS) Excerpta Medica. International Conference Series 513.

47. Medical Research Council (1973) Responsibility in the Use of Medical Information for Research. *British Medical Journal* 1 213-6.

48. Inman, WHW. (1980). Post-marketing surveillance of adverse drug reactions in general practice. Part I. Search for New Methods. Part II Prescription-Event Monitoring at the University of Southampton. *British Medical Journal* 282.1131-2. Ibid 1216-7.

49. Inman, WHW. (1985). Let's get our act together. *Side-Effects of Drugs Annual* No 9. MNG (ed) Dukes. Elsevier, Amsterdam.

50. XVth International Rheumatology Congress (1981). *European Journal of Rheumatology and Inflammation*. 5.2.

51. Inman, WHW. Risks of Medical Intervention in, Cooper MG.(ed)(1985) *Risk: Man-made hazards to Man*. Wolfson College 1984. Oxford University Press 1985.

52. Rothschild (1978). *The Listener* 30th November.

53. Venning, GR. (1983). Identification of adverse reactions to drugs. *British Medical Journal*. 286.199-202:289-292:458-460:544-447.

54. Inman, WHW. (1983). Adverse Reactions to New Drugs. *British Medical Journal*. 2 86.219-720.

55. Delmothe, T (1989). Drugs Watchdogs and the Drug Industry. *British Medical Journal*. 299, 476.

56. House of Lords Select Committee on the European Communities. (1991). The European Medicines Agency and Future Marketing Authorisation Procedures. HMSO London.

57. Inman, WHW. (1988). Blood disorders and suicide in patients taking mianserin or amitriptyline. *Lancet.* 90-92.

58. Dukes, MNG. (1990). The van der Kroef syndrome. *Side Effects of Drugs Annual 1990.* Elsevier. Amsterdam.

59. Waller, PC., Wood, SM., Langman, MJS., Breckenridge, AM. and Rawlins, MD. (1992) Review of company postmarketing surveillance studies, *British Medical Journal.* 204: 1470-72.

60. Erlichman, J (1987). *Guardian* Sept 9th.

61. Inman, WHW. (1989). PMS and 'Brass Tacks' in RD Mann (ed) Risk and Consent to Risk in Medicine. Parthenon Publishing Group.

62. Drug Safety Research Unit (1988). PEM News No 5.

63. INCA Newsletter Winter Issue 92/93.

64. Inman, WWH. and Pearce, G. (1993). Prescriber profile and post-marketing surveillance. *Lancet.* 342.658-61.

65. Gill, P., Scrivener, G., Lloyd, D. and Dowell T. (1995). The effect of patient ethnicity on prescribing rates. Health Trends 27: 4. 111-3,

66. Hansard [Lords] 28 April 1993 249-382.

67. Association of the British Pharmaceutical Industry (1995) Guidelines for company-sponsored safety assessment of marketed medicines (SAMM). ABPI Data Sheet Compendium 1995-96 xxvii-xxix.

68. Lynn, M. Sunday Times 10th November 1996.

Abbreviations

AAH	Allied Anthracite Holdings - Meditel
ABPI	Association of the British Pharmaceutical Industries
ADROIT	Adverse Drug Reactions On-line Information Tracking
APVDC	Association of Parents of Vaccine-Damaged Children
ASLEF	Association of Locomotive Engineers and Firemen
BCDSP	Boston Collaborative Drug Surveillance Program
BDC	British Dyestuffs Corporation.
BMA	British Medical Association
BSE	Bovine Spongiform Encephalopathy
CFCs	chlorofluorocarbon compounds
CJD	Creutzfeld-Jakob Disease
CNS	central nervous system
CSD	Committee on Safety of Drugs (Dunlop Committee)
CSM	Committee on Safety of Medicines
DHSS	Department of Health and Social Security
DSRU	Drug Safety Research Unit
EE	ethinyloestradiol (a component of oral contraceptives)
FDA	Food and Drug Administration (USA)
FPA	Family Planning Association
GMSC	General Medical Services Committee (of BMA)
HIPE	Hospital In-patient Enquiry
HPT	Hormone Pregnancy Test
IBM	International Business Machines
ICI	Imperial Chemical Industries Ltd
ICL	International Computers Limited
ICP	Imperial Chemical Pharmaceuticals Ltd
IMS	Intercontinental Medical Statistics Ltd
INCA	Integrated Network for Computer Administration
JCVI	Joint Committee on Vaccination and Immunisation

KIKADIS Kyoto International Conference Against Drug-Induced Sufferings
LA   Licensing Authority (of DHSS)
MCA   Medicines Control Agency
ME   mestranol (a component of oral contraceptives)
MRC   Medical Research Council
NDA   New Drug Application
NHS   National Health Service
NSAID   Non-Steroidal Anti-Inflammatory Drug
OPCS   Office of Population Censuses and Surveys
PEM   Prescription-Event Monitoring
PPA   Prescription Pricing Authority
PQs   Parliamentary Questions
PMS   Post-Marketing Surveillance
PTMO   Part-time Medical Officer
SAMM   Company-Sponsored Safety Assessment of Marketed Medicines
SMON   Subacute myelo-optico-neuropathy
SCV   Subcommittee on Complications of Vaccination (of JCVI)
UHFH   Unexplained Hepatitis Following Halothane
VAMP   Value Added Medical Products
WHO   World Health Organisation

Index